SalonOvations' Staffing Policies & Procedures

&a &a &a

Page
142

91

SalonOvations' Staffing Policies & Procedures

by Beverly Kilmer

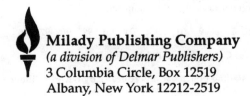

Milady Publishing Company
(a division of Delmar Publishers)
3 Columbia Circle, Box 12519
Albany, New York 12212-2519

NOTICE TO THE READER

Publisher does not warrant or guarantee any of the products described herein or perform any independent analysis in connection with any of the product information contained herein. Publisher does not assume, and expressly disclaims, any obligation to obtain and include information on other than that provided to it by the manufacturer.

The reader is expressly warned to consider and adopt all safety precautions that might be indicated by the activities herein and to avoid all potential hazards. By following the instructions contained herein, the reader willingly assumes all risks in connection with such instructions.

The publisher makes no representation or warranties of any kind, including but not limited to, the warranties of fitness for particular purpose or merchantability, nor are any such representations implied with respect to the material set forth herein, and the publisher takes no responsibility with respect to such material. The publisher shall not be liable for any special, consequential, or exemplary damages resulting, in whole or in part, from the readers' use of, or reliance upon, this material.

Cover Design: D. Dupras
Cover Photo: Brian Yacur

Milady Staff
Publisher: Catherine Frangie
Acquisitions Editor: Marlene McHugh Pratt
Project Editor: Annette Downs Danaher
Production Manager: Brian Yacur

COPYRIGHT © 1996
Milady Publishing
(a division of Delmar Publishers)
an International Thomson Publishing company I(T)P

Printed in the United States of America
Printed and distributed simultaneously in Canada

For more information, contact:
SalonOvations
Milady Publishing
Columbia Circle, Box 12519
Albany, New York 12212-2519

1 2 3 4 5 6 7 8 9 10 XXX 01 00 99 98 97 96

Library of Congress Cataloging-in-Publication Data
Kilmer, Beverly.
    SalonOvations' staffing policies & procedures / by Beverly Kilmer.
        p. cm.
    Includes index.
    ISBN 1-56253-314-2
    1.Beauty shops — Personnel management. 2. Beauty shops — Employees —
Recruiting.   I. Title.
TT965.K55   1996
646.7'2'0683—dc20   95-52680
                                                                        CIP

Contents

About the Author

Beverly Kilmer is the founder of the United Salon Owners' Association, the president of National Alliance of Salon Professionals, and an experienced salon owner. She is dedicated to helping salon owners achieve maximum success and is tireless in her enthusiasm for professionalism for all beauty professionals. For the past three years she has registered as a lobbyist in order to demand greater standards for the beauty profession. She is a highly sought, high-energy workshop and seminar leader, trainer,. and speaker.

Her past experience as owner of three salons has given her the insight and expertise to write this book. While admitting there are no guarantees to a problem-free salon environment, Beverly feels that by taking the philosophies of her book to heart, salon owners will greatly increase their likelihood for staffing success.

Acknowledgments

First and foremost, I want to thank Marlene Pratt at Milady Publishing Company, for not letting me turn this opportunity down. She knew if I really wanted to do this book, I'd find the time. And she was great at allowing me the flexibility I needed. I want to acknowledge the fact that most of my knowledge has come from attending seminars, reading books, and being obsessed with the need to learn from others. There is no way that I could possibly list every individual who has helped make this book possible. But I will say that if you wrote a book on salon or business management, I have read it. If you gave a seminar on salon or people management, I was there. If you spent even a few minutes talking with me, you are responsible in part for this book. This book is the result of my experience as a salon owner and the experiences of hundreds of people I have come in contact with through the years. And to all of them I will be forever grateful.

Also the publisher would like to thank the following professionals for their time and expertise in reviewing this manuscript: Patty Ferraro, Boca Raton, FL; Karen Sasnett, Tallahassee, FL; and Lenny King, Longwood, FL.

Introduction

Salon staffing remains by far the most difficult responsibility facing salon owners today. There are no short cuts or magic formulas to being a great boss or manager. Your stylists probably will not grow old with you. You will have many employees coming and going over the years. It will often be like a virtual roller coaster ride and many times you will feel like it is taking place in the middle of a tornado where you have little or no control.

This book is designed to give you that control. It will help you understand what motivates and encourages staff members to give their best to you, your salon, and the clients that patronize your salon. It will help you know when to hire and how to better utilize the staff you have. You will learn to focus on making the right decisions when hiring and realize that panic hiring never works.

You'll develop a new understanding of the four personality types and how each interacts with the other. You'll know during the interview if that prospect will be able to fill your salon's needs and if you will be able to satisfy the needs of the applicant, which is equally important.

This book deals with the topics of knowing when to hire, holding a successful interview, finding reliable employees, and being able to offer not just a job, but a career building position with growth and long-term potential. You'll also learn what to do to keep your employees once the hiring is done, how to encourage unity and teamwork by empowering your staff to be a part of the decision making process, and how to establish effective salon policies and procedures that reflect positive attitudes and work for the betterment of all concerned.

This book may not solve all your staffing problems, but it will enable you to make better decisions based on a new understanding of your own needs and those of the people around you. Sound business decisions as opposed to emotional decisions will win out every time.

Chapter 1

Finding, Keeping, and Growing with Your Staff

The Salon Owner's Prayer

Now I lay me down to sleep
I pray, oh Lord, my stylists I'll keep

And as we go from day to day
Please help them always want to stay

I'll work hard to help them see
How very special and important they are to me

But should they decide to spread their wings
Help me to wish them only the best of everything!

by Beverly Kilmer

INTRODUCTION

Throughout the United States, staffing remains the salon owner's number one challenge. With dramatic changes taking place in the salon industry, owners are finding themselves facing more difficult and complex situations every day. The costs of locating, hiring, and training employees have consistently risen over the past several years. Across the country, salon owners are caught in the middle of a war with no apparent winners.

However, there are solutions to all of life's challenges, including the compensation dilemma. By gathering as much information and knowledge as possible, the successful salon owner is able to stay abreast of the changes. This allows the owner to make more educated and profitable decisions. In this chapter, I will take you through the many stages of locating, hiring, and retaining qualified, efficient, and long-term staff members.

WHERE HAVE ALL THE STYLISTS GONE?

Whenever I meet with a group of salon owners, I always hear the same thing: "There are no stylists out there," or "I run ads in the paper and get no response." The situation is the same throughout the country.

Before you make the effort to locate the elusive stylists, take time to analyze honestly your past hiring techniques, your management strengths and weaknesses, the reasons your former employees left your salon, your actual need for additional staff, the skills required, and your salon's atmosphere and personality. Take an objective look at your salon, and ask yourself if you would want to work there. List five things that you absolutely love about your salon and five things you would change. List the benefits of working for you.

5 THINGS I LOVE ABOUT MY SALON

1. _____
2. _____
3. _____
4. _____
5. _____

5 THINGS I WOULD CHANGE ABOUT MY SALON

1. _____
2. _____
3. _____
4. _____
5. _____

THE BENEFITS OF WORKING IN MY SALON

1. _____
2. _____
3. _____
4. _____
5. _____

Let's analyze your past experiences one by one.

Faulty Hiring Techniques

Very often, owners tell me they are at a loss as to why the stylists they interview choose not to take the job. "Why don't they want to work for me? I have a beautiful salon and I do everything for my staff. I just don't understand."

I'm sure you've heard the saying, "If it sounds too good to be true, it usually is." Too often, salon owners are so excited to have a potential stylist within their grasp that they engage in "overkill." Working so desperately to convince the stylist that their salon is heaven on earth, the owners not only never give the stylist the opportunity to talk and ask important questions, but they literally talk him or her out of taking the position.

Hiring practices can determine success or failure for a salon. Many times desperate owners, in a state of despair, proclaim, "At this point, I just need a warm body." This approach to staffing is a single-ingredient recipe for immediate failure. Panic hiring has never been effective for anyone. The new hire grasps the feeling of power immediately. Salon owners who hire in a state of panic find themselves not in control, but being controlled.

Effective Hiring Techniques

The following techniques are effective in hiring quality stylists:
- Use the employment application as a springboard for successful hiring.
- Ask the right questions at the interview.
- Read between the lines of the application.
- Check references.
- Know specifically what you are looking for in a stylist.
- Determine to hire a stylist whose career path looks like it was designed for the beauty industry.

The Interview and Application

Use the employment application at the interview to zero in on quality stylists whose skills and experience are right for your salon. Is the application completely filled out? This is an indication of efficiency and organizational skills as well as the ability to complete a task. Did the stylist list the requested past employment information and references? It is important to know a stylist's past salon experiences. You should *always* check with past employers. If it isn't feasible to contact the most recent, then contact the previous employer.

Doing these things will benefit not only you, but everyone involved in your salon. You have a responsibility to yourself, your salon, your existing staff, and your clients to hire responsibly. Everyone in your salon, including yourself, should enjoy going to work.

Chapter 2 provides an example of a salon application for employment. You can have it printed as is with your logo or modify it to meet your needs. The important thing is to allow the application to work for you. It can be and should be your most powerful hiring tool.

Recruiting

There are many things you can do to recruit quality stylists and cultivate contacts even if you don't have an immediate hiring need.

- In all your display ads in magazines, newspapers, TV, radio, and billboards, place a statement that your salon is always accepting applications from talented, career-oriented stylists.

- Exercise ongoing involvement with local schools. Not only will this allow you to get to know the students, but you will have the opportunity to help them become more work ready. You can invite potential graduates to visit your salon as observers. The more time they spend with you and your staff, the more likely it is that they will join your team.

- Literally everyone you know has a hair stylist. Send the word out through friends, neighbors, and acquaintances that you are looking to establish, increase, or enhance your salon team. With many people recruiting for you, your salon will be staffed in no time at all, or it will be enhanced with quality stylists when you need a replacement or addition.

- Purchase a list of licenses from your state licensing board. Send a tasteful cover letter to stylists on that list. Outline your salon's benefits and your requirements, and include a salon brochure or menu.

Understanding Your Management Strengths and Weaknesses

Some people are natural managers, leaders, and motivators. Others are not. Successful salon owners recognize their managerial strengths and weaknesses and make adjustments. The following are common management weaknesses:

ɞ Salon owners who work behind the chair as a stylist 10 to 12 hours a day cannot manage their staff.

ɞ The extremely sensitive "I want to be your friend" salon owner cannot make consistent, objective business decisions.

ɞ The quick-tempered "It's my way or the highway" salon owner tends to alienate everyone sooner or later.

ɞ The prima donna, who needs to be the star of the salon, does not encourage individual professional growth for staff members and will ultimately chase everyone away. By nature, we all want the opportunity for advancement. When there is nowhere else to go, the stylist will eventually go somewhere else.

If you possess any of these traits, you should hire a salon manager and relinquish the duties that require strengths you do not possess. The ideal manager will handle staffing situations in an objective, unbiased, and professional manner. You will be involved only from behind the scenes. You will be aware of the issues and can make recommendations, but the manager is responsible for the day-to-day staffing interactions.

Evaluating Past Staffing Problems

It is important to analyze immediately why an employee left your salon. It is impossible not to take it personally when an employee leaves. However, this happens to everyone sooner or later. If you can learn from it and prevent the loss of your remaining staff, then it can become a win-win situation for everyone.

Encourage the exiting stylist to explain, in detail, why he or she is leaving. If the stylist is uncomfortable about doing so, ask him or her to send you a letter explaining his or her reasons for leaving.

Talk with your remaining staff and reassure them that you understand their concern and that you are open to suggestions that will help lead to a smoother running workplace. As soon as possible, carefully encourage discussion of the ex-employee. Try to be alert to staff members' comments and mannerisms. Most of all, learn from the experience and allow something good to come from a traumatic situation. Correct the mistakes of the past.

Determining Your Hiring Needs

Many owners believe that if they have six chairs, they must put six people behind them immediately, regardless of potential clientele. Having too many stylists and too few clients can be disastrous. Unless you have serious walk-in potential, you shouldn't try to build or book more than one stylist at a time. As each stylist approaches a 65% consistent book, then it is time to hire the next stylist.

Two or more stylists with little to do will usually spend a lot of time sitting around talking about how your salon doesn't have any business. It is much better for salon morale if you add staff members as you need them. Everyone will be happier, busier, and wealthier: again, a win-win situation.

Ask yourself the following questions when you consider your hiring needs:

1. Do you have sufficient clients to warrant additional staff? One rule of thumb for determininig when to hire additional staff is the productivity level of your salon. You will want to have a productivity level of at least 65% before you hire another staff member without his or her own clients. First you need to establish your salon's potential productivity level. You use the following formula to do so: hours open per week _____ × number of chairs _____ × potential productivity = _____. Then you must establish your salon's actual productivity, using the following formula: total salon hours booked per week _____ ÷ potential productivity _____ = actual salon productivity rate _____ %.

For example, if your salon is open 40 hours per week and you have four chairs, you have the potential of 160 booked or potential chair hours. To establish your actual booked hours, divide your actual booked hours by your potential booked hours. This will give your actual salon productivity rate.

You will need to decide when the productivity warrants additional staffing. It is always important to have existing staff members happy and content. Idle hands lead to negative thoughts and backroom gossip (usually about the salon's lack of business). You don't want to add to that scenario. It is much better to work on building a strong client base and build a need for additional staffing before hiring. Getting and keeping good people is easier if they are actually needed. If your ad is going to read "Stylist with clientele needed for busy salon," you might want to rethink your needs. You are really saying that you need *clients* but will also accept a stylist.

2. What areas of service are understaffed? Again, it is very important to hire for your needs. If you are a chemical-directed salon, you will want to hire someone with chemical experience or have them work in an assistant or training program. It is extremely dangerous to hire a new stylist and let him or her do color and perming right away. These are the most complex of all the services offered in a salon, as well as the most financially rewarding. By hiring the right person, your chemical business can skyrocket. The same holds true for cutting, styling, nails, skin care, etc. Decide what your needs are and hire the solution to that need. The result will be a win-win situation for everyone, especially the client.

3. Are you able to departmentalize? If your salon is large enough to departmentalize, you will be able to emphasize the need for specialists. Even if your salon is a two- or three-chair salon, you can still have departments such as chemical, artistic/styling, cut-

ting, make-up/facial, and nails. Each department needs to receive special attention and be treated as a separate profit center. By treating it as such, it immediately becomes responsible for constant growth and for making a profit. Everyone likes to feel important and have the opportunity to shine. By hiring the right person to act as department head of each service center in your salon, you will be guaranteeing salon growth, stylist satisfaction, and client delight.

4. What kind of employee are you really looking for? You are looking for top performers—the top 10%. Ninety percent of employees are lazy, undependable, shop hoppers, and instigators. You are looking for the other 10%. How do you find them? By asking for them. Send out the right message with a well-conceived ad describing the degree of expertise you are looking for and what you have to offer. Advertise that you are offering a position, not just a job. That position carries with it a lot of responsibilities. However, only top performers are qualified. Here is a partial list of the traits present in top performers:

Self-starter	Anxious to help others
Enthusiastic	Gutsy
Optimistic	Technically skilled
Positive attitude	Success driven
Nondefensive	Enjoys a challenge
Take charge, go-getter	Financially motivated
Action oriented	Emotionally motivated
Professional	Visionary
Loyal	Pride in self and others
Strong people skills	Gets along well with coworkers
Personally focused	

It is not always easy to recognize superstars, and there are no sure-fire guarantees. However, by learning to understand yourself and your own personality traits, it will be much easier to recognize and manage others. Recognizing body language and the art of reading people will be your best hiring tool.

✿ RECOGNIZING BEHAVIORAL TYPES

There are four basic behavioral types of people:

Dominant(D)   Influencing (I)   Steady (S)   Cautious (C)

Each of the four types has a different way of seeing the world and communicating with others. By understanding the basic-differences of each type, you will be able to communicate more effectively.

Dominant Personalities

Traits of dominant personalities

- Direct
- Results oriented
- Decisive
- High ego
- Dominant
- Impatient
- Driver
- Original

- Impulsive
- Critical
- Self-assured
- Inquisitive
- Realistic goals
- Self-Reliant
- Sometimes blunt
- Demanding

Wants of the D

- Freedom
- Quick results
- Authority
- Prestige
- Direct answers
- Opportunity for achievement

- Independence
- Varied activities
- Competition
- Power
- Changes

Fears of the D

- Being taken advantage of
- Slowness
- Not being taken seriously
- Being too jovial
- Loss of control
- Not being influential
- Being too soft
- Inaction
- Boredom

To be effective, the D needs

- To develop empathy
- To be a better listener
- To relax
- To pace self
- Deadlines
- To keep busy
- To be organized
- Challenging assignments
- To pay attention to details
- To be more tactful

How the D behaves with others

- Enjoys confrontation
- Limits personal contact
- Bored with routine
- Can be manipulative
- Likes change
- Impatient
- Stick to business at hand
- Responds quickly
- Displays competence

How to deal with a D

- Limit small talk
- Build his or her ego
- Avoid details
- Be prepared
- Respond quickly
- Stick to the issues
- Be patient
- Give freedom to grow

The D Cosmetologist

D cosmetologists can be great motivators, energizers, educators, salon coordinators, managers, and team leaders. They want to do a good job and be recognized for their efforts. They often look for recognition over financial rewards (but not for long). In hiring a

D for a position of power, be sure to take into consideration the prima donna tendencies and ego traits that are a factor with Ds. By being aware of these traits and using them to your salon's benefit, hiring a D can be a major plus for any salon. One thing to keep in mind is that you cannot change a D. If you are a D, it is important for you to consider the needs of the D. If you are aware of the areas that you need to be conscious of, you will find yourself relating to the needs of your staff in a more positive manner. It is true that you can't change a D; however, you can be aware of how others react to your actions.

The best way to handle a D is to give him or her a job with responsibility, growth potential, changeability, and a job deadline. Ds get restless very easily and are constantly looking for a way to express themselves. Ds also make great platform artists and can be used to train new staff members, as well as existing staff. You should always take advantage of the high energy level of a D. With proper understanding and handling, a D can be a tremendous asset in your salon.

Influencing Personalities

Traits of Influencing personalities
- Socially poised
- Promoter
- Optimistic
- Articulate
- Image oriented
- Impulsive
- Persuasive
- Trusting
- Disorganized
- Influential
- Verbal
- People oriented
- Positive
- Enthusiastic
- Team player

Wants of the I
- Recognition
- To look good
- To persuade
- Money
- Favorable working conditions

- To be optimistic
- Freedom of expression
- To work with others

Fears of the I

- Loss of approval
- A fixed environment
- Using a hard sell
- Being alone
- Details
- Taking advantage of people

To be effective, the I needs

- Time control
- To be more organized
- Tangible rewards
- Others who can follow through
- Others with a logical approach
- Awareness of impact on others
- To take on fewer tasks at one time
- Technical knowledge
- To be more patient
- Emotional control

How the I behaves with others

- Eager to talk
- Optimistic
- Shows self-confidence
- Works well with others
- Dislikes conflict
- Praises others
- Tends to exaggerate
- Entertaining
- Great persuader
- Open with ideas
- Difficult to keep on schedule
- Very people oriented

How to deal with the I

- Be personal
- Allow him or her to verbalize
- Keep directed
- Be encouraging
- Give space
- Stay on schedule
- Don't dwell on details

- Encourage creativity
- Give an audience
- Give praise and recognition

The I Cosmetologist

The I cosmetologist is fun to be around. He or she is easily excitable and anxious to try new techniques and styles. The I is the first one to wear a new color or cut and is often viewed as the salon trendsetter. Because I cosmetologists are very people oriented, they usually take initiative in building a clientele by letting acquaintances know what they do and encourage their business. The I is rarely shy about asking for business. Clients tend to be extremely loyal to the I personalities due to their like-able and optimistic nature. Everyone likes to be around people who make them feel good, and I cosmetologists are feel-good people who make great morale builders in the salon.

The I cosmetologists can be annoying at times, however, by being manipulative, impulsive, and displaying behavior that is inappropriate for certain situations. They often engage in salon gossip or accidentally break confidences of co-workers. This is usually not premeditated; it is merely a result of letting the mouth engage before the brain kicks in. The I cosmetologists never intentionally hurt anyone; it is simply a lack of thinking first. The I has a disregard for detail and is usually in a hurry. Because of this, I cosmetologists are often inconsistent in their quality of work, giving a beautiful cut this month and not being able to duplicate it next month. The I personality reflects the 80-20 rule: Success is 80% people skills and 20% technical skills. It is important for this personality to maintain very good client records and review them as a refresher before seeing the client.

When hiring an I, be sure you have the client base, or walk-in traffic, to sustain an additional employee. I cosmetologists tend to be hyper and are not good at sitting. If the business is not there, the I won't be patient for long. As stated earlier, I cosmetologists will do their part in building a clientele; however, they do expect to be busy relatively soon. Unfortunately, the I cosmetologists are often the shop hoppers. You have to work at keeping them happy and satisfied. However, it is worth the effort. They sell big ticket services and lots of retail, because they like money!

When issues arise that require a reprimand or criticism, do so in a helpful and caring manner. Loud and abusive approaches will always backfire with the I, who is very emotional and is offended easily.

The I cosmetologists make great employees, especially in an enviroment that allows and encourages creative expression and freedom.

Steady Personalities

Traits of steady personalities

- Stable
- Possessive
- Loyal
- Consistent
- Team player
- Passive
- Supportive
- Family oriented
- Steady
- Predictable
- Patient
- Disciplined behavior
- Good listener
- Can hold grudge

Wants of the S

- Stability
- Credit for achievements
- To own things
- Organization and structure
- Conflict-free environment
- Group membership
- Admiration
- Independence
- To be in control
- Time to think and plan

Fears of the S

- Loss of financial security
- Change
- Disorganization
- Uncontrolled emotions
- Challenge
- Dependence on others
- Conflict
- Risk of any kind
- Antagonism
- Crowds

To be effective, the S needs

- Time to adjust to change
- Personal attention
- Friendship
- Guidelines
- Encouragement
- Others who react quickly
- Independence
- To be asked rather than told
- Reassurance
- Facts and figures
- Confidence in others
- To be in control

How the S behaves with others

- Steady and predictable
- Empathetic
- Modest
- Extremely dependable
- Asks a lot of questions
- Tries to please
- Logical
- Loyal
- Good listener
- Good work habits
- Noncompetitive
- Avoids conflict

How to deal with the S

- Provide a conflict-free environment
- Allow to work at own speed
- Give trophies, plaques, rewards
- Praise publicly
- Don't surprise
- Give details and related information
- Be patient
- Show sincere interest
- Don't challenge or pressure
- Don't expect quick decisions

The S cosmetologist

The S makes the most loyal employee. The S wants approval and won't take part in backroom gossip. S cosmetologists are not shop hoppers. They do not like change and will usually stay with a salon for years unless they are backed into a corner or made to feel that they are not wanted. They can hold a grudge if they feel they have been wronged, and in such a case you will have to work very hard to make amends.

The S personality is very conscientious and always wants to please. S cosmetologists are very caring of their clients and do extra things for them. They take great pride in doing a good job and will usually take longer to do a service because they require perfection of themselves.

The S personalities operate better in a structured environment with policies and procedures. They like to know what is expected of them, and they expect others to abide by the rules as well. People usually tell all their troubles to the S, and the S can be extremely discrete, never disclosing any secrets or confidences bestowed on them. The S cosmetologists are usually on time for appointments. They like to have control over their bookings and don't like to work appointments in while working on a client. They get nervous knowing a client is waiting on them. They do not work well under pressure.

Cautious Personalities

Traits of cautious personalities

- Perfectionist
- Avoid risk
- Accurate
- Sensitive to criticism
- Data oriented
- Logical thinker
- Sincere
- Conscientious
- Detail oriented
- Great listener
- Well prepared
- Accommodating of others
- Avoid conflicts
- Analytical

Wants of the C

- Time to think
- A plan
- High standards
- Time to research details
- No pressure
- Minimal risk
- Security
- Explanations

- Stability
- Friends

- Family
- Reassurance

Fears of the C

- Criticism of work
- Loss of control
- Serenity
- Rapid change
- Confusion
- Instructions

- Antagonism
- Losing
- Conflict
- Not being liked
- Irrational acts
- Loss of financial security

To be effective, the C needs

- To be encouraged
- Strong support
- Precision work
- Self-confidence
- Relaxation methods
- Security

- Appreciation
- Success experiences
- Facts with which to make decisions
- Organization

How the C behaves with others

- Suspicious
- Reserved
- Detail oriented
- Aloof at first

- Friend for life
- Overly sensitive
- Can't say no
- Wants to do for self

How to deal with the C

- Provide an abundance of data
- Show appreciation and respect
- Prove yourself

- Offer a stable workplace
- Avoid criticism
- Be accurate
- Ask, don't demand
- Be a friend

The C Cosmetologist

The C cosmetologists are the most analytical of all personalities. They are the most distrusting. However, once you win their trust, it is for life. The C is easygoing and unassertive, overly sensitive, and easily bullied. The C is quiet and withdrawn and is not considered a people person. However, Cs are willing to do anything for anyone. They are the first people to help in a crisis situation. The Cs are level headed and make decisions on the facts only, not on emotions. They do not like phonies.

The C is very loyal once a friendship is formed. Cs are hard to get to know and are often considered aloof. It is harder for Cs to build a clientele. However, they take great pride in the quality of their work and always deliver quality. Once they win a client over, it is usually for good. The Cs want to work in a well-organized atmosphere. They want the salon owner to have control and to correct problems in the salon. If problems aren't addressed, the C will usually look elsewhere for work.

The C makes a good take-charge person. Cs don't worry about being liked; they attend to business and are concerned with the bottom line. When you prove your loyalty to them, they will be loyal to you. They are extremely honest.

Chapter 2

Hiring and Dehiring

 INTRODUCTION

"I can't find good stylists who want to work." "When I do find good stylists, as soon as they start paying off for me, they leave." Sound familiar? You bet it does! We've all heard it and most of us have said it. While there are no easy answers, it will help immensely if you decide who you need in your salon. Know what your needs are and remember, *Don't panic hire!* It never works out.

It is a good idea to have an employment ad running often, even when you aren't in need of a stylist. Keep a current stock of applications on file at all times. Scrutinize the applications closely and make notations so that you will know, at a glance, who you are interested in hiring. Above all, be ethical when hiring. Remember the golden rule: "Do unto others as you would have others do unto you." It doesn't read "Do unto others before they do unto you." In addition, never call a potential employee at work in another salon. Calling is fine, but not at the salon.

When hiring, don't fall into the trap of feeling forced to offer higher commissions. You know what you can afford. Be strong and stick to it. If you pay more than you can afford, you will quickly come to resent paying the higher percentages and never feel good about your new hires. It is unlikely that this working relationship will be able to survive the resentments and strains.

❀ IDEAS FOR RECRUITING

The following ideas will help you recruit quality stylists:

- Talk to other salon owners and exchange applications. (Someone you did not hire may be perfect for the salon down the street, and vice versa.) Networking pays off!
- Talk to your staff and other stylists you know. Happy, satisfied employees offer the same word-of-mouth advertising as happy, satisfied clients. Encourage your staff to let friends know the advantages of working in your salon.
- Give your business card to someone you see who has an attractive style. Ask her to give it to her stylist.
- Do a mailing to all licensed stylists. State your benefits.
- Be involved with your local beauty schools.
- In your salon display ads, have an announcement that your salon is always accepting applications for professional, career-oriented stylists and nail technicians (or whatever your needs may be).
- Sell yourself at beauty shows. Attending local educational programs is a great way to meet career oriented stylists. Take advantage of this opportunity to pass out your business card.
- The perfect recruiting ad paints a clear picture of who you are, what you are offering, and who you are looking for.
- There are advantages to hiring both new and experienced stylists. The new stylist comes eager to learn and is more likely to adjust to your salon's policies. They are more motivated by education and encouragement than the experienced stylist.

The experienced stylist is usually very confident, capable, and able to produce from day one. However, they may bring unwanted habits from previous salons, and may be motivated by money as opposed to education and the vision of growth.

Just as important as finding good employees is keeping them. The best way to ensure long-term employees is to be prepared when hiring. Know what you are looking for and settle for nothing less. Talent and technical ability are great, but optimism and enthusiasm are essential. Ability can be learned, but enthusiasm comes from within.

Consider your clientele when hiring. If your salon caters more to college-age people, you are far better off to hire younger, more progressive stylists. If you are in a conservative area, hiring very young stylists with avant-garde hairstyles and clothing and no knowledge of curler sets and tease styles, could be disastrous. You should know your clientele and hire accordingly.

An issue that needs to be addressed is the fact that, in all likelihood, you are not going to grow old with your employees. The industry average for a stylist's stay in one salon is two and a half years. Some may stay longer, but the majority will not. Acceptance of this could be the beginning of a whole new way of life for you. Enjoy your staff while they are with you and wish them well when they choose to move on.

As a salon owner, it is up to you to set the atmosphere and attitudes in your salon. Set your standards, have written policies, and stick to them. Have all new recruits read and sign a copy of the policies that govern your salon.

WHEN IS IT TIME TO LET GO?

For some reason, salon owners rarely fire employees. They are afraid of losing clientele and revenue. Why let bad employees destroy your salon morale and risk losing other productive stylists by keeping them when you know the relationship is not working? You know it is not working, the stylist knows it, and you can bet the clients know it. The stylist will leave sooner or later and will take clients and revenue away from your salon. In addition, the stylist will talk bad about you and your salon after leaving. Why should you keep such employees on your payroll while they are destroying your creditability among your other employees and clients? Every day you allow them to come to your salon, you are allowing them to do you more damage and you are paying them to do it to you.

USING THE APPLICATION TO FIND QUALITY STYLISTS

The employment application is more than a piece of paper: It is a tool that, if used properly, can help you hire top-quality people and avoid the hassle of hiring a person who is not right for your salon and having to fire him or her later. The following example of an employment application is effective in hiring quality stylists.

Application for Employment

Personal

Last Name First Middle	Date
Street Address	Home Telephone
City, State, Zip	Business Telephone
Have you ever applied for employment with us? ❑ Yes ❑ No If yes, Month and Year _____ Location _____	Pay expected
Position Desired	When will you be available to begin?
Can you attend evening meetings and/or classes? ❑ Yes ❑ No Can you attend morning meetings and/or classes? ❑ Yes ❑ No Can you work evenings? ❑ Yes ❑ No	Employment Desired: Full Time ❑ Part Time ❑

Professional

(Please check applicable spaces)

1. Are you experienced in hairdressing? _____ Skin Care _____ How long? _____

2. Are you a recent beauty school graduate? _____

3. Have you worked for a nonappointment salon? _____ How long? _____

4. Special needs: Hours ____ Child Care ____ Transportation ____ Holidays ____ Insurance ____

5. I want to know about: Training _____ Benefits _____ Vacation _____ Advancement _____

Years of experience _____ Areas of specialization _____

Do you have a Cosmetology license in this state? ❑ Yes ❑ No

Have you regularly attended any manufacturers' clinics or seminars? ❑ Yes ❑ No   Which? _____

How do you rate yourself as a hairdresser? ❑ Excellent ❑ Very Good ❑ Average ❑ Fair ❑ Poor

Rate the top 5 salon services you perform in order of your preference. Mark your favorite "1," your next favorite "2," etc.

☐ Cutting   ☐ Conditioning   ☐ Coloring   ☐ Styling   ☐ Other

☐ Perming   ☐ Manicuring   ☐ Skin Care   ☐ Makeup   _____

Education

School	Name and Location of School	Course of Study	No. of Years Completed	Did you graduate?	Degree or Diploma
College				☐ Yes ☐ No	
Business/Trade/Technical				☐ Yes ☐ No	
High School				☐ Yes ☐ No	

Salon Employment

(1)

Salon Name	Telephone ( )
Address	Employed (State month and year) From To
Name of Supervisor	Weekly Pay Start Last
State Job Title and Describe Your Work	Reason for Leaving

(2)

Salon Name	Telephone ( )
Address	Employed (State month and year) From To
Name of Supervisor	Weekly Pay Start Last
State Job Title and Describe Your Work	Reason for Leaving

(3)

Salon Name	Telephone ( )
Address	Employed (State month and year) From To
Name of Supervisor	Weekly Pay Start Last
State Job Title and Describe Your Work	Reason for Leaving

Other Employment

(4)

Company Name	Telephone ( )
Address	Employed (State month and year) From To
Name of Supervisor	Weekly Pay Start Last
State Job Title and Describe Your Work	Reason for Leaving

References

Please list three references (include at least two professional references).

Name _____ Phone (_____) _____
Address _____
City _____ State _____ Zip Code _____
Title and/or relationship _____

Name _____ Phone (_____) _____
Address _____
City _____ State _____ Zip Code _____
Title and/or relationship _____

Name _____ Phone (_____) _____
Address _____
City _____ State _____ Zip Code _____
Title and/or relationship _____

You are required by the Immigration Reform and Control Act of 1986 to complete Form I-9 within three business days of being hired. If you are hired by this company, you must complete the form and show acceptable documentation according to Immigration and Naturalization Service guidelines. Compliance is a condition of employment.

I hereby verify that all the information I have provided on this job application is true and correct to the best of my knowledge.

Signature_____Date _____

Additional Questions That May Be Included on the Application

The following questions can be used on an employment application to give you a more detailed, personal picture of the potential employee.

If you need more room to answer the questions below, use the back of the sheet.

1. Describe the perfect work situation. _____
   _____

2. Describe the perfect boss. _____
   _____

3. What do you expect to get out of working here, and what can we expect to get out of you?
   _____
   _____

4. How do you expect the salon to help you build a clientele?
   _____

5. What steps do you plan on taking to build your clientele?
   _____

6. Would taking early or late appointments present a problem for you?
   _____

7. How do you feel about assisting? _____
   _____

8. Describe what teamwork means to you. _____
   _____

9. List your three strongest assets._____
   _____

10. Why are you changing jobs? _____
    _____

After Reviewing the Prospect's Application

By using our application or one that is similar, you will be able to make a more informed judgment as to whether the prospect would suit your salon's need and, just as importantly, you will be able to fulfill the prospect's expectations. The questions associated with this application are designed to have the prospect give insightful answers as to their long-term ability to perform the responsibilities of the stylist position. By analyzing the answers, you will know without a doubt whether you want to hire or not.

It is best to review the application in depth after the interview and if you are impressed by the interview, the appearance of the prospect, and the application responses, you may find the perfect stylist. At this point, you will want to hold a second or third interview and make your offer.

You need to evaluate the prospect in view of his or her likelihood for long-term employment in your salon. The following tips will help you do so:

❧ Rely on your instincts. Often, you will have a gut feeling that the person will not work out, but you need to hire someone right away so you ignore the warnings Listen to your inner feelings and at least analyze why you might be hesitant. Doing so could save you months of working through a bad situation and possibly losing other good employees.

❧ Ask yourself if your salon will be able to offer the prospective employee what he or she is seeking. It is easy to offer the moon in order to encourage a prospective employee to come and work in your salon. But it never pays to offer what you cannot deliver. Remember, it is always better to underpromise and overdeliver, especially with your staff. Be honest about what you can deliver in terms of pay, benefits, education, and working conditions, and be honest about your expectations.

❧ Think about the needs of your salon. Is the prospective employee really going to be able to perform according to the standard and technical needs of your salon? Does he or she fit your salon's image? Will the prospective employee fit in with your other staff members? Teamwork is extremely important for any successful salon. What is this person's reputation? Has he or she previously been stable and not been a shop hopper? What do you think are his or her leadership qualities and career goals? Are they consistent with your own?

After analyzing these issues, you should be ready to make a qualified decision to hire or not to hire the prospective employee.

 ## SIGNS OF TRUE LEADERSHIP

When people feel good about themselves, motivating them comes naturally. Having high self-esteem helps people relate better to those around them. They are not worried about what other people are thinking about them, and their salon owners or managers will benefit from their self-confidence. These people are not only great employees, but they also act as motivators for the rest of the staff.

Here are some ideas that will help your staff members feel better about themselves:

- Give your undivided attention when staff members talk to you. This will show them that you care about them and what they have to say.
- Give staff members responsibility and let them do it their way. Let them follow a task through all the way, even if they are doing it different from what you would have suggested. They may actually have a more effective way, and you will reap the benefits.
- When conflicts arise among co-workers, allow them room to resolve the problem without interference, whenever possible.
- Don't be afraid to express your feelings, especially the good feelings.
- Allow and encourage your staff to express their feelings.
- Admit when you make a mistake.
- Immediately make the effort to correct your mistakes.

- Look for the good in each employee every day and you will find it.
- Never miss the opportunity to praise or reward positive efforts.
- Avoid putdowns, especially in front of co-workers.
- Express trust and respect for staff and co-workers.
- When a reprimand is necessary, make sure the employee's act is the disappointment, not the employee.
- Allow the staff to be a part of the decision-making process.
- Don't expect employees to perform services they are not thoroughly trained to perform.
- Never show favoritism. This will always backfire on you.
- Set your salon's standards and rules. Be consistent in enforcing them.
- Never expect your staff to live up to standards that you are not willing to live up to every day of your life. Don't ask of them what you would not be willing to do yourself.

SEEING IS BELIEVING

Too often the problems in a salon are not caused by actual occurrences, but by the staff's or owner's perception of the problem. There are often discrepancies in the way staff members and owners perceive situations. Consider the following comments of owners and staff members:

What the owners are saying about the staff

- They never take any initiative around here.
- They just don't care about the kind of work they do.
- Why should I keep trying, they don't seem to care what I do for them anyway?
- When you ask them for their ideas and what they want, they never give a straight answer.

- If you give them an inch, they'll take a mile.
- I have to treat them like I'm their mother. They can't do anything on their own.
- I'm tired of their petty complaints.
- They want to make more money, but they don't want to take extra clients or be more available when clients want them.
- When we have a meeting, I let them know what I expect and they all agree, but then they do just like they were doing before.
- If only I could find good help who want to work.
- Stylists don't know anything. They come out of school and I have to teach them how to hold the scissors.
- Why can't I keep stylists? They never stay in one salon for more than a year or so, just long enough to get clients and then they leave.
- They just don't realize how lucky they are to be working in a salon like this. No other salon would give them everything I do.
- I'm always available for them to come talk to me about anything, but no one ever does. They would rather talk to each other in the backroom.

What the staff members are saying about the owners

- They don't care about us and our problems.
- I wish they would listen to what I have to say. If this was my salon, I would . . .
- How can they be so dumb!?
- They never have the products I need when I need them.
- They are always acting as if they are afraid for us to know what is going on. It's like they think they have a secret.
- They say one thing today and another thing tomorrow. I never know what is expected.
- They never listen when I try to tell them what is bothering me, and then they act as if they are surprised.

- I just come in and do my job. I'm not going out of my way for them anymore. They don't care about me, so why should I make money for them?
- I try not to rock the boat.
- Every meeting is the same. We will be yelled at for everything that has gone wrong for a month—as if it's all our fault.
- Before she bought this salon, she was fun and we were friends. That was why I came with her to this salon. And now all she does is push me to do more clients, fold towels, and sweep the hair. Nag, Nag, Nag!
- They are always complaining about money, but I see what they are making. They are making a lot of money off all of us and they want us to feel sorry for them. Ha!
- I'm supposed to retail product, but they never have what my clients want and I'm not gonna sell them something else. If they don't stock it, I am not going to retail.

When making the decision to hire staff, take a few minutes to remember when you were seeking employment as a stylist. What were your thoughts during the interview, your first week as a new employee, and later when you were considering finding a new job or opening your salon? Role playing is one of the best forms of reality checking. Make a concerted effort to avoid all the factors that discouraged you as an employee. Find good people, hire them, and work like the devil to keep them.

THE CUSTOMER CONCEPT

You should consider your staff just as important as, if not more important than, your clients. In essence, your staff is your internal customer. Staff members should be sought after and nurtured just as a valued client would be. Replacing a client is much less expensive than a stylist. Lets look at the numbers: a client spends a total of $650 annually in your salon. With her family, let's assume that you receive a grand total of $1200. That is a lot of money to lose. To replace her, you run an advertisement special in the paper. This costs you $125 plus a $15 discount for the service she gets. She will be back, however, for future services, and you have just replaced the client you lost earlier at a cost of only $140. That's not too bad.

However, the costs are much higher when a stylist leaves. She takes all of her clients with her. You run an ad to find a new stylist. You run the ad for a minimum of five days ($225) but usually as long as a month or more. The average stylist generates approximately $500 per week. This equals $2000 per month plus at last $225 for the cost of the ad.

Positive customer service begins with the people who work for you. Hiring for longevity means being committed enough to be selective. There are certain things you need to take into consideration when preparing to hire:

❧ Treat each vacancy like your future depends on it. It does! Define the responsibilities of the position. Consider both the people skills and the technical skills equally in the decision to hire.

❧ Decide ahead of time what skills are needed for the position and settle for nothing less. Your standards must be met. Your reputation is on the line. Don't allow your reputation to be placed in less than professional hands.

❧ Ask meaningful what-if questions. Ask questions and listen to the meaning of the answer, not just the words. Remember, you can learn a lot more from listening than from talking. Some meaningful questions you might want to ask are as follows:

> ❖ What does giving the client good service mean to you?
> ❖ Give me an example of when you gave exceptional service.
> ❖ Since you have been here, what have you noticed that we are doing that is good or needs to be improved?
> ❖ We all get discouraged from time to time when dealing with people. What do you do to keep yourself up?

❖ How do you handle difficult clients?

❖ What do you like most about the beauty profession?

As you have noticed, these are all people-directed questions. The first issue you want to address is people skills. To have a future as a beauty professional, you must have a love of people. To ensure that the stylists you hire have good people skills, try the following:

- Invite the prospect to visit your salon for a day to become familiar with your salon's personality, your staff, and the type of clientele your salon services.
- Encourage the prospect to analyze you and your salon as well. Potential employees must be comfortable in your salon to be effective for you and for themselves.
- Consider searching for staff in all the unlikely places. Literally everywhere you go is an opportunity to recruit. The checkout person at the grocery has her hair done by someone. Don't miss an opportunity to let people know your salon has an opening.
- Recruit actively, always. Good employees may not know where to find you. Where did you find your best people? There may be others there who are looking for a new home.
- Set your standards. First rate hires first rate.

Chapter 3

Holding a Successful Interview

 INTRODUCTION

The hiring process is a critical factor in any business, but especially in the beauty profession. This is such a personal and possessive industry that hiring the wrong employee can lead (and often has led) to the fall of many potentially successful salons.

The wrong stylist can not only cost you valuable clients, but can turn a previously content salon staff into one of low morale, discontent, and even rebellion. This can happen so fast that you don't realize what is going on until it is too late and you are faced with a massive walk-out. This not only affects your internal salon operation, but it severely affects your salon clientele.

Always remember, you can learn more from listening than from talking. Plan and outline your interview thoroughly. First impressions are just as important from the prospect's view as from yours. You need to appear in control, extremely organized, and self-confident.

By understanding the four personality traits discussed in Chapter 1 and having a better knowledge of people's hot buttons, motivators, fears, and needs, you can better choose the staff members that are likely to be long-term assets for your salon.

◈ SUCCESSFUL INTERVIEW GUIDELINES

Interviews are critical to the entire working relationship between employer and employee. First impressions are important not only to the employer: The message the prospective employee receives can set the tone for what he or she perceives is expected. In addition, prospective employees will decide, at that first meeting, if they feel the employer is an effective manager.

Be alert to your first impressions. They are often right on target. During the interview, be conscious of your good language as well as that of the prospect. The message you send during the interview will last long after you have made the decision to hire. If you allow the prospect to do the interviewing, you will be viewed as not in control and over-eager to hire. This is **not** the message you want to send.

You will want to ask questions that encourage the prospect to do the majority of the talking. You want to know as much about him or her as possible. Don't ask yes/no questions; instead, ask open-ended questions.

Choosing the right people for your salon is an important responsibility that should always be taken seriously. As stated earlier, never panic hire. It is important to make sure that all employees are compatible. Tension in the salon is a sure way of losing clients and perhaps your better stylists as well.

A good interview isn't difficult to do. By taking time to prepare for the interview, you will save hours of training time and retain clients that might have been lost by hiring the wrong stylists. The interview is intended to give the prospective employee and employer an opportunity to exchange information about each other and the salon.

Things You Should Know about Your Applicant

- ❧ Their work history. Find out as much about their work history as possible. By all means, do check references.
- ❧ Their career plans. Find out where this person is headed. Find out if your effort in training him or her is justified. Someone

who is definitely headed for another career and is just filling in time is not a good prospect for your training efforts and expenses.

🙠 Their expectations of you. Know what this person is expecting from you. Be honest. If you cannot deliver what is expected, admit it. The time to face this is before you hire someone. You don't want to have a reputation for not delivering the goods.

Things Your Applicant Should Know About You

🙠 Salary, compensation, and benefits. Everyone wants to know what is in it for them. This especially holds true for employees. Leave nothing to chance. Don't promise benefits you are not able to deliver. If it is possible, however, do offer some form of benefits package. In this time of employment insecurity, it is important to offer benefits.

🙠 Hours required to work. Let the applicant know the salon hours, and discuss the times you will be needing coverage.

🙠 Salon image and clientele. It is *most* important that your stylists be accommodating to your clientele. This means hiring according to the needs of your clients and being sure the applicant is aware of the type of work needed. Your employees must fit the image that you have chosen for your salon.

🙠 Discipline. Don't be afraid to discuss your salon standards and the method of handling issues as they surface.

Remember, what you say or don't say at an interview is just as important as what the prospective employee is saying. Before the interview, plan what to say and what to ask. But even more importantly, take time during the interview to listen intensely.

Let's Interview!

QUESTIONS FOR THE APPLICANT

It's time to start with the question segment of the interview. Asking the right questions can make all the difference. Ask questions that allow you to read between the lines. Many applicants will answer straight questions the way they think you want them answered. You want to ask questions that let you know how the applicants really feel and what you can expect of them. Start by asking questions that will get the applicant talking about experiences in the salon environment. There is a wealth of information in this kind of information. Often, this is all you will need to make your decision, although we do not recommend you stop here.

The following can elicit the kind of information you need:

1. Tell me about the most interesting client you have ever had.
2. What type of client gets on your nerves? How do you respond to this client?
3. What do you like best about the beauty profession?
4. What do you dislike most about the beauty profession?
5. What service do you wish you never had to do again, and why?
6. What would you like to see changed about our profession, and how could it be changed?
7. Why did you enter this industry, and how far do you expect to go in it?
8. Describe the perfect salon environment.
9. What kind of advertising do you think works for a salon?
10. Why do you want to change jobs?
11. What motivates you?
12. How do you expect to improve your career at our salon?
13. What kind of contribution do you plan to make to our salon?
14. Do your clients buy salon or drug store products?
15. What products do you use at home?
16. Why do your clients come back to you? What do you do that's special?
17. Do your clients usually book their next appointment at their current appointment?
18. Why should I hire you for this position?

19. Describe the perfect boss.
20. Tell me about the perfect day in the perfect salon.

By listening to the applicant and letting him or her elaborate on the topics listed, you will have enough information to make a responsible decision about whether he or she would be an asset to your salon. Just as important, you will know if you can deliver what the applicant is anticipating. The hiring should be a positive career move for both parties.

During the interview, you should be alert to the affirmative action guidelines that dictate what you are not allowed to ask. This information can be obtained from your state Department of Labor office. Improper questions can land you in hot water and in the middle of a lawsuit, so avoid any questions relating to race, religion, sex, political affiliation, children, marital status, financial status, and especially age.

Have your questions prepared in advance and ask all the applicants the same questions. Do not prequalify an applicant and omit the interview on the basis of an applicant's appearance. Even if this is a dead give-away that you would not hire that person, you must follow through with the interview if it was scheduled.

STATEMENT OF YOUR NEEDS

By now you know how much farther you want to go with the interview. If you are not interested in hiring this applicant, give a brief overview of your salon and what you are looking for in an employee. Tell the person you will review his or her application, and get back in touch if interested. If you are feeling good about this applicant, you will want to make him or her aware of your salon's philosophy, organizational structure, and job descriptions. (These will be discussed in depth in Chapter 4, "Salon Policies and Procedures Guidelines.") You don't want to have any surprises once the new employee is hired. If everyone knows what to expect from the beginning, you will have less discontentment within your salon.

The philosophy is important because it outlines your mission, vision, and standards. When you decided to open your salon, it was your dream. You had distinct ideas of how you wanted your salon to look, the way clients would be treated, and the people who would be working for you. Don't lose sight of your dream. The people you hire must be willing to buy into your philosophy or you will quickly lose sight of your dream and your salon will become just a place where people do hair, nails, or skin care.

The organizational structure of your salon outlines how each department of service in your salon is set into motion and who is responsible for its success. By organizing the structure of operation in your salon, your staff members can perform their jobs in the most efficient manner. The organizational structure is a picture of how each employee's job fits into the framework of your salon's vision, mission, and standards. The so-called chain of command is identified in the organizational structure, and each person knows to report to the person next on the ladder. By developing a good structure, each person will know and understand the team structure and their own responsibilities as a team member. This is the foundation of a powerful team salon. (See Figure 3.1.) Everyone working for you should know the person they are to answer to and who can help them when they have questions or need assistance.

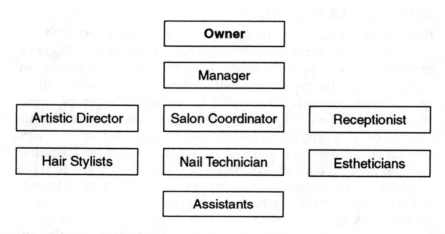

Figure 3.1 Example of a salon organizational chart.

Job descriptions let everyone know exactly what their duties are. Winning is achieved by knowing the rules and playing to win. Every position in your salon should include a job description, regardless of what the job is. Even the cleaning person, who comes in to clean for you once a week, needs a description of exactly how you want the floors mopped, waxed, or swept, and how you want other cleaning tasks handled.

A job description should include job qualifications, job duties and responsibilities, and quality standards for the job. Job qualifications specify the requirements necessary to acquire the position. Job duties and responsibilities outline the responsibilities of the position. This tells the employee what needs to be done in order to complete the job. Quality standards ensure that you have total control of your dream. Everything relating to your salon should reflect the standards you have established for your salon. Your standards become the basis for evaluating your staff's efficiency and performance.

Assuming that you and the applicant are mutually agreeable to the applicant joining your team, this would be a good time to introduce him or her to your salon policies and procedures. This can be done at this meeting or postponed until a second interview session.

Chapter 4

Salon Policies and Procedures Guidelines

 INTRODUCTION

To be an effective manager or employer, the staff you hire must be aware of what is expected of them. Your staff can and should be your most valuable asset. However, if you do not hire, train, and nurture your employees in the most effective way possible, your staff quickly becomes a liability.

By developing and implementing your own policy and procedures manual, you are establishing your salon as a well-organized entity with definite standards. Too many salons fail to set standards of any kind. They feel that their salon does have high standards, but they fail to delineate them. However, standards, like goals, must be written to be effective. No one can read your mind and know what is expected. You must have and use written business plans, salon goals, and staff retention plans. All of this translates into the use of a well-prepared policy and procedures manual.

⬛ OUTLINE FOR A PROCEDURES MANUAL

On the following pages you will find an extensive, in-depth outline for developing your own customized policy and procedures manual.

How to Use this Guideline

1. First review the entire outline.
2. Make notes of issues that should be discussed with staff.
3. Include staff input when making an initial draft of guidelines.
4. Establish the policy and procedures manual and stick to it. The latter is the more difficult but most important factor.
5. Remember the importance of stability and consistency. Enforce the policies of your salon consistently, once they are established. By doing so, you will gain the respect of your staff by showing them your dedication to your salon, as well as their own success.
6. Give each member of your staff a copy of the policy and procedures manual.
7. Have new hires sign a form of acceptance that they have received, read, and agree to abide by the policies of your salon. This form should go in their employee file.
8. Remember that the policy and procedures manual protects both the staff and management. Use it with that in mind.
9. Remember that by implementing these guidelines, you are guaranteeing your clients and staff the best possible salon atmosphere.

Salon Policy and Procedures Outline

1. Name, address, and phone number of salon
   A. Hours open
   B. Days open
2. Name of salon owner

3. Mission and vision statement describing the goals and philosophy of your salon (It is important for your staff to share in your mission and vision. Not only do they need to know what your mission and vision is, they need to know how they fit into them. For employees to help you reach your goals, they need to feel as though doing so will help them reach their goals as well. This needs to be a mutually beneficial voyage.)

4. Statement of purpose for the policy manual (A policy and procedures manual must have a purpose. Specify exactly what you expect to gain from the use of the policies you've outlined.)

5. Salon image and personality (This is where you share your dream—what sets you aside from the crowd, and what you want clients to see and feel when they walk in the door.)

   A. Salon history

   B. Salon appearance

   C. Salon atmosphere

6. Employee etiquette (These are the standards you expect your staff to live up to—the way they will handle situations on a consistent basis. Anything that goes in this category is a must, and you should give a lot of thought to establishing these guidelines.)

   A. Code of professionalism

   B. Personal appearance, dress code, conduct, and attitude

   C. Guidelines for client relations and retention

   D. Team spirit and interaction

   E. Staff meeting attendance requirements

7. Job descriptions—duties and responsibilities (Outline the responsibilities of each position you have available. Be consistent in your expectations. Take time to analyze each job individually and how you would like to see the job performed. Put yourself in the place of the client and go through the entire visit. The job description should reflect what it takes for the client to receive exceptional service, not just satisfactory service.)

A. Owner

B. Manager/salon coordinator

C. Stylist

D. Nail technician

E. Technical assistant (shampoo, chemical, etc.)

F. Make-up artist/facialist/esthetician

G. Receptionist

8. Employment qualifications for all positions (List the minimum qualifications you will allow in an employee and then look for much more in an applicant.)

9. Advertising and public relation policies (Outline your advertising procedures. List the process you will use in bringing clients into the salon, as well as the way in which you will be building name recognition for your salon.)

10. Pricing structure for services and retail (Employees need to know how to charge the client. It is awkward if a new employee must ask constantly what to charge a client. It is also uncomfortable for the client.)

11. Product lines used and sold in the salon

12. Client handling policies (Not only should all of the areas mentioned in this section be included here, but you should have a training session for all new employees as well to reinforce client handling policies. This is an area that needs consistency above all others. Every client that comes into your salon should be treated with excellent service every time by all employees. All problems should be addressed in the appropriate manner, and everyone should be clear about what the appropriate manner is.)

A. Client's first visit

1. How clients will be distributed

2. Use of client card files

3. Handling of consultations

B. Client complaints

C. Techniques for regaining and retaining lost clients

13. Appointment book policies (This is another very important

area that needs intense training. Front desk operations can make or break a salon without anyone knowing what went wrong. Set your policies in stone.)

A. Scheduling appointments

B. Prebooking appointments

C. Obtaining phone numbers

D. Providing add-on services

E. Handling cancellations

F. Confirming appointments

14. Compensation (This is the "what's in it for me," Everyone wants to know your compensation program and how it is set up. This should be explained at the initial meeting, when you hire new employees. Don't have different pay systems for different people unless you have a specific pay scale structure that applies to everyone. Employees do discuss paychecks, even when they say they don't. You can't play favorites when it comes to money.)

A. Salary

B. Bonus structure

C. Retail incentives

D. Benefit package

   1. Vacation

   2. Holidays

   3 Sick days

   4. Insurance

   5. Employee discounts

   6. Servicing family and friends

E. Educational policies

   1. New-hire training

   2. Advanced education

   3. In-salon training

15. Departmental positions (If you are departmentalized, outline the responsibilities of each position. This is an excellent way of growing the different profit centers of your salon.)

16. Evaluations and reviews (State how often you will be doing evaluations, who will be doing them, and the areas in which staff will be evaluated. Let it be known that evaluations are done for the purpose of helping your staff expand their career goals. Evaluations should be positive reinforcement in any salon.)

17. Work schedules (This lets the staff know the hours they will be required to work. If evening and weekends are required, the employee should know this when being hired.)

18. Lunch and break policy (By law, everyone is entitled to take lunch and periodic breaks. This needs to be listed in your policy. If staff members choose to work through lunch, it is a good idea to have a disclaimer in their employee file that they have requested the options of working through lunch. The labor boards of most states are concerned with employers not allowing lunch breaks. It important to comply with all state and federal labor laws.)

19. Acceptable and unacceptable absence (Outline exactly what your policy is concerning absenteeism. Document absences in employee files.)

20. Tardiness (Again, outline your policy. You never know when you will need documentation.)

21. Working outside the salon (Employees should be aware of any restrictions you may have on their outside employment.)

22. Monetary pay procedures (This is another area for which you should be very conscious of the long-term consequences. State your policy and stick to it. Outline how you will handle each of the following situations.)

    A. Cash advances

    B. Check handling—Pay period
        1. When is payday
        2. For what period (date to date)
        3. Retail compensation or pay

    C. Cash register shortage or overage

    D. Tipping policy

23. Gossiping in the salon (It is a given that gossiping will not be tolerated in any way. **State this in your policy in bold-face type.**)
24. Salon maintenance and cleanliness (List who is responsible for this, as well as how and when it will be done.)
25. Telephone policy (Outline what will be tolerated and what will not. Put yourself in the client's place when making this decision.)
    A. Procedures for answering
    B. Etiquette
    C. Personal phone calls
26. Smoking policy
    A. Clients
    B. Staff
27. Discipline policy and procedure (Outline the procedures that you will follow. Any action at all, even verbal, should always be notated in employee files.)
28. Termination policy (List the actions that would necessitate termination. Remember, you must have valid reasons such as theft, detriment to business, etc., to fire someone. You should have at least three written reprimands on file for an employee to be released. Be aware of the labor laws in your particular state, as well as the federal labor laws.

Salon Policy and Procedures Outline: Worksheet

1. Name, address, and phone number of salon

   Name _____

   Address _____

   Phone number _____

   A. Hours open _____

   B. Days open _____

2. Name of salon owner

   Owner _____

3. Mission and vision statement describing the goals and philosophy of your salon

   _____

   _____

   _____

   _____

4. Statement of purpose of the policy manual.

   _____

   _____

   _____

5. Salon image and personality

   A. Salon history

   _____

   _____

   _____

   B. Salon appearance

   _____

   _____

   C. Salon atmosphere

   _____

   _____

   _____

6. Employee etiquette

   A. Code of professionalism

   _____

   _____

   _____

B. Personal appearance, dress code, conduct, and attitude

_____

_____

_____

C. Guidelines for client relations and retention

_____

_____

_____

_____

_____

_____

D. Team spirit and interaction

_____

_____

_____

E. Staff meeting attendance requirements

_____

_____

7. Job descriptions—duties and responsibilities
   A. Owner

_____

_____

_____

B. Manager/salon coordinator

_____

_____

_____

C. Stylist

_____

_____

_____

D. Nail technician

_____

_____

_____

E. Technical assistant (shampoo, chemical, etc.)

_____

_____

_____

F. Make-up artist/facialist/esthetician

_____

_____

_____

G. Receptionist

_____

_____

_____

_____

8. Employment qualifications for all positions
   A. Manager/coordinator

_____

_____

_____

B. Stylists

_____

_____

_____

C. Nail technician

_____

_____

_____

D. Technical assistant

_____

_____

_____

E. Make-up artist/facialist/esthetician

_____

_____

_____

F. Receptionist

_____

_____

_____

_____

9. Advertising and public relation policies

_____

_____

_____

10. Pricing structure for service and retail

_____

_____

_____

11. Product lines used and sold in the salon

_____

_____

_____

_____

12. Client handling policies
    A. Client's first visit
        1. How clients will be distributed
        2. Use of client card files
        3. Handling of consultation

_____

_____

_____

_____

_____

_____

_____

_____

    B. Client complaints

_____

_____

_____

_____

    C. Techniques for regaining and retaining lost clients

_____

_____

_____

_____

13. Appointment book policies

  A. Scheduling appointments

  _____

  _____

  _____

  _____

  B. Prebooking appointments

  _____

  _____

  _____

  _____

  C. Obtaining hone numbers

  _____

  _____

  _____

  D. Providing add-on services

  _____

  _____

  _____

  E. Handling cancellations

  _____

  _____

  _____

  F. Confirming appointments

  _____

  _____

  _____

14. Compensation
    A. Salary

    _____
    _____
    _____
    _____

    B. Bonus structure

    _____
    _____
    _____

    C. Retail incentives

    _____
    _____
    _____
    _____

    D. Benefit package
       1. Vacation

    _____
    _____
    _____
    _____

       2. Holidays

    _____
    _____
    _____
    _____

       3. Sick days

    _____
    _____
    _____
    _____

4. Insurance

_____

_____

_____

_____

5. Employee discounts

_____

_____

_____

_____

6. Servicing family and friends

_____

_____

_____

_____

E. Educational policies
   1. New-hire training

_____

_____

_____

_____

   2. Advanced education

_____

_____

_____

_____

   3. In-salon training

_____

_____

_____

15. Departmental positions

_____

_____

_____

_____

_____

_____

_____

_____

16. Evaluations and reviews

_____

_____

_____

_____

_____

_____

_____

17. Work schedules

_____

_____

_____

18. Lunch and break policy

_____

_____

_____

_____

19. Acceptable and unacceptable absence

_____

_____

_____

20. Tardiness

_____

_____

_____

21. Working outside the salon

_____

_____

_____

22. Monetary pay procedures
    A. Cash advances

    _____

    _____

    _____

    B. Check handling—Pay period
        1. When is payday
        2. For what period (date to date)
        3. Retail compensation or pay

    _____

    _____

    _____

    _____

    _____

C. Cash register shortage or overage

_____

_____

_____

_____

D. Tipping policy

_____

_____

_____

23. Gossiping in the salon

_____

_____

_____

_____

24. Salon maintenance and cleanliness

_____

_____

_____

_____

25. Telephone policy
    A. Procedures for answering

_____

_____

_____

B. Etiquette

_____

_____

_____

C. Personal phone calls

_____

_____

_____

26. Smoking policy
    A. Clients

_____

_____

_____

    B. Staff

_____

_____

_____

27. Discipline policy and procedure

_____

_____

_____

_____

_____

_____

28. Termination policy

_____

_____

_____

_____

_____

_____

29. Brief summary

_____

_____

_____

_____

_____

_____

_____

_____

Chapter 5

Staffing Your Salon With Love

INTRODUCTION

Choosing the right people for your salon is an important responsibility that should always be taken seriously. Again, never panic hire. There is a fine line between staffing your salon and stuffing your salon. A warm body is not better than nobody.

It is imperative that all staff members be compatible. Do your homework *before* you hire. Ask the right questions, as mentioned earlier, and be sure to follow through with checking references and getting feedback from existing staff members. Once you have made your decision and have hired new staff members, follow the guidelines discussed in this chapter to ensure that your salon runs smoothly.

THE ALL IMPORTANT EARLY WEEKS

How you handle the first few weeks of a stylist's employment is extremely important. Your new stylist is excited and eager to start his or her new career with your salon. This is a time for establishing your strength as a professional. You must use your managerial skills on an ongoing basis. You cannot be all things to all people. However, what you can and should be is a source of security and stability throughout the salon. Everyone wants to know that his or her work environment is secure and that the salon will still be there next week.

Acceptance from fellow workers is one of the most critical factors in the first few weeks for most new employees. If there is antagonism among workers, everyone—including clients—will suffer. Take pains during hiring procedures to ensure that everyone is compatible. In addition, when you make the decision to hire new employees, your existing staff should be aware of that fact. They should never learn it from the applicant as he or she calls for an interview.

The more successful salons are now offering a mentor program within the salon. This serves several purposes. It involves the current staff in the hiring process and helps create a bonding environment between staff members. By assigning a new hire to a more experienced staff member, you will be allowing the current staff to feel a part of the new hire's success. It is a win-win for everyone.

 ## PATIENCE, PERSISTENCE, AND PRAISE

The beauty industry is probably the most egotistical of all professions. Stylists are artistic, temperamental, independent, and, of course, wonderful. Dealing with these personalities sometimes demands a powerful dose of managerial patience.

The smart salon owner will work hard to reinforce the strengths of his or her staff members. Salon owners should never feel threatened by employing dynamic stylists. The more dynamic the staff members, the more dynamic the salon. This will ensure a very successful business for all concerned.

Rewarding good work and achievements is as necessary as breathing in today's salon world. Everyone wants to be recognized and appreciated.

The key to retaining good staff is consistency. Today's salon owners should learn to maintain an even, flowing personality regardless of the moment's trials and tribulations. Even the most strict salon owners can be, and usually are, respected and appreciated as long as they are consistent. It is important to discipline, praise, and operate daily on a consistent basis so that everyone knows what to expect.

How and When to Praise

Praise is one of the most effective motivators. Be generous with praise when it is deserved. Too often the power of praise is overlooked. Praise openly, but professionally. Don't overdo it. By all means, be sincere. There is little worse than phony praise. It actually does more harm than good. Your body language will give you away. (A rule of thumb: If you don't mean it, don't say it.)

How and When to Scold

Unfortunately, if you own a salon you will occasionally have to scold or reprimand someone. The key is to be diplomatic and consistent. Keep in mind that you are doing so for the good of your employee as well as the good of your business and its clients. When correction is necessary, by all means, do it in private. Always meet staff with a private and positive focus. Encourage individual and professional growth as long as it doesn't endanger your salon business in any way.

 BASIC TRAINING

There should always be an ongoing training program in your salon. No one is ever overtrained. Education is a major issue in the success of any salon. Education comes in many forms, such as salon classes and classes given by manufacturers, local educators, or even your own staff members. (Everyone has talents to be shared with others when encouraged.) There are also distributor shows and manufacturer shows.

As just mentioned, magic can happen in your own salon when you utilize the talents you have in-house. Take advantage of your own "show-quality" people. Allow your own staff members to share knowledge and education at staff meetings. Hold hair clinics and shows for your clients. The extent of available education is limited only by your lack of creative forces.

Basic training not only encompasses technical training, but also people skills. Technical skills are of little value without people skills. Communication is invaluable in the beauty industry, which is the ultimate people business. Communicating is not only speaking, but also listening and giving body language and signals. Very often, what you do speaks louder than what you say. A smile or a frown tells it all.

Training within the salon has got to come in many forms and to serve many purposes. Success needs to be gauged by advancements in productivity and progress of the staff. You and your staff will need to establish goals that are challenging and achievable. Everyone needs something to work towards. If you are not moving forward, you are moving backward. There is no such thing as sitting still in business.

By establishing an in-salon continuing education program, you will be assured that your staff and salon will be moving forward. Success comes through the continued advancement of one's goals.

THE BEGINNING STYLIST

Many salon owners want to hire stylists with clientele. However, this is the real world. More stylists are moving around less. This is viewed as both good news and bad news, depending on who you are talking to. Thus, it is becoming both necessary and smart to hire newly graduated stylists. The drawbacks, however, are as follows:

- They don't have a clientele, so they are going to cost you money for a while.
- They are inexperienced, so you are going to have to spend time training them.

On the other hand, the advantages are as follows:
- They are eager to learn.
- They haven't established so-called bad habits.
- You have the opportunity to mold them into top-notch, highly motivated professional stylists.
- Since you are instrumental in building their clientele and, in essence, their career, the stylists tend to be more loyal.

The beginning stylist should work in conjunction with an experienced stylist—preferably with someone confident enough to train a new recruit. For growth purposes, it is advantageous to assign management positions as they come available to your qualified staff members. These could include, but are not limited to the following:

- Chemical director or manager
- Skin care specialist
- Nail care director or manager
- Staff director
- Retail and operations manager

DEALING WITH TOO MUCH ENERGY AND AGGRESSION

Have you ever met someone who was so full of positive energy that he or she literally made you tired just being in the same room with him or her for an hour? This type of person may irritate you in day-to-day life, but that same energy, when channeled in the right direction, can mean big money to your salon. You can utilize positive staff energy by having such people do the following things:

- Teach and share with other staff members.
- Promote the salon at civic functions and other outside functions.
- Develop in-salon promotions.
- Be a team leader, motivator, etc.

Occasionally, stylists get bored and will use their energies in a negative way that can damage staff morale. When you hire stylists, let them know that you will not tolerate such behavior. If you know a stylist tends to encourage negativity when bored or restless, plan ahead to keep this person busy in a positive way. Negativity breeds negativity. Remember, one negative person can bring down 10 happy people. However, 10 happy people cannot bring up one negative person.

This leads us to negative aggression, which is a salon owner's nightmare. Stylists who engage in negative aggression usually find fault with everything and everyone in the salon, including the clients. The negative stylist almost always has little, if any, self-confidence and feels threatened by co-workers.

The negative personality is extremely difficult, if not impossible, to change. If co-workers are understanding and tolerant of the aggressive stylist, then you have a chance of turning the person around by building on his or her positive traits. This will be a long-term project, but if everyone agrees that the person can be a valuable asset, and if everyone is willing to work together, it may be worth the effort. The important factor is not to jeopardize your better employees in order to retain a problem employee.

DEALING WITH JEALOUSY

Jealousy is a common problem in the beauty industry because, as stated previously, this is a very egotistical business. Most people keep their jealousy under control, but a few let it interfere with their job and co-workers. Jealousy can't be allowed if it becomes a problem with co-workers or clients.

Sometimes stylists are jealous of the salon owner. Salon owners can dismantle this situation by encouraging employee self-esteem and helping employees realize how valuable they are to the salon and its owner.

Another form of jealousy is that of a stylist and his or her clients. Few things upset a stylist more than stopping by the salon on a day off and seeing one of his or her clients in the chair of another stylist. This is an issue that needs to be outlined in your policy and procedures manual. Feelings cannot be dictated, but attitude expression can and should be addressed.

DEALING WITH THEFT

This is a topic we all wish did not have to be discussed. Unfortunately, such is not the case. Most likely, theft will have to be addressed in your salon. Depending on your inventory control procedures, it is usually easy for your staff to steal from you. This is not to say that the theft is intentional. A lot of unplanned theft takes place in most salons. Consider the following examples of innocent and dishonest theft.

Innocent or Unintentional Theft

> ๛ A stylist is out of hair spray at home and, as she is headed out the door and remembers that the register is closed out, she just grabs her half-empty can off her station, planning to bring it back the next day. Of course, she forgets.

- A stylist's mom needs a perm and can't come to the salon. The stylist asks to borrow one of your perms and replace it when she goes to the supply house. She forgets to do so.

These are true examples of people who do want to replace or pay for the products they've borrowed, but they forget. We live in such a fast-paced world that it is hard for us to remember to pay an electric bill, much less pay for a $5.00 perm.

Dishonest and Premeditated Theft

- You don't have an effective inventory control, and everyone knows it. A stylist assumes that you won't miss one bottle of shampoo or conditioner. Once he or she gets away with this, you become the supplier of all his or her hair care needs.
- A stylist becomes a cash drawer thief. However, your cash drawer is your livelihood. You should always be able to trace every transaction that takes place in your salon on any given day, at any given time. This is your responsibility to yourself, your staff, and your business.
- A stylist gives the client one price and actually reports another. This is very common, and all salon owners and managers should implement a system that does not allow for a stylist to quote different prices without first clearing them with management. Thousands of dollars are lost per year in any given salon due to individual pricing.

Theft should not be tolerated under any circumstances. If you have proper inventory control and strong management policies, theft is less likely to occur in your salon.

RIGID OBEDIENCE

Rules and regulations are necessary and even desired by most staff members. However, it is possible to be too rigid and unbending. There are usually two sides to every issue, and the salon is no exception. There is the staff's view, and there is management's view. Salon owners often assume that since they own the salon, what they say goes. If only it were that easy, everyone would own a salon. Instead, policies and procedures must be a matter of what is best for all concerned—the staff, the owner, the client, and the salon business. By addressing most issues during the hiring process and utilizing your policy and procedures manual, you will eliminate many discipline problems. In addition, you must consider the views of staff members when problems arise. Communication is still the master of success for everyone.

SELLING YOUR STAFF ON CHANGE

Salon owners often lose the support of their staff in compensation changes because they
- Don't show them the incentives necessary to increase their profits as well as the salon owner's.
- Don't give staff enough information to understand the entire compensation package, such as benefits, payment scale, education, etc.
- Don't involve staff in developing the new compensation structure.

The best way for an owner to sell a compensation changeover to the staff is
- By realizing that the words *take away, remove,* and *deduct* will have a negative impact on the staff and can only serve to block a compensation change right from the start.
- By explaining the positive aspects of a changeover in terms of rewards for productivity and incentives for growth.
- By creating an encouraging atmosphere that will allow employees to develop a heightened sense of self-worth and job security.

- By educating staff on an ongoing basis in regard to the importance of recognizing the essentials of good business, which are not just technical skills.
- By giving the staff some input into how the overall system will be developed. Remember, systems don't work on their own. People make systems work.

It is important for salon owners to accept that no matter how the change is presented, there will be some who will not be in favor of it. It is unrealistic to expect every person to accept a compensation change.

The owners who are most successful at making the change in compensation are those who try to understand the point of view of staff members. Stylists' most frequent objections are as follows:

- The stylist is used to being paid a certain way and is now suspicious of a new way being better.
- There is a lack of stylist input into the new system.
- The owner has a "take it or leave it" attitude.
- Too little time is given for making the transfer.
- There is a lack of total understanding of the new system.
- There is a lack of unity among stylists and the owner.
- There is a lack of communication on the owner's part.
- The owner lacks interest in staff feedback.
- Staff members suspect that they are getting the short end of the stick.
- Change comes too quickly for the staff to adjust to the change.

Stylists are more likely to accept a compensation change and welcome it if they feel that their needs are being fulfilled. They will be satisfied with the change when

- They realize that the traditional system is being restructured in favor of a more modern system.
- They see that the new system offers incentives, growth, and security.

- They see that fringe benefits are a different form of salary.
- They realize that a high commission doesn't guarantee a high take-home pay.
- They realize that the salon's programs are roads to increasing their personal earning potential.
- They understand that in a competitive market, good business principles can mean excellent earnings.
- They see that they can't have it both ways—high commission plus benefits.
- They want incentive programs and recognize their value.
- They believe the new system will result in more opportunities to increase take-home pay.

Chapter 6

Building Unity Within the Salon

 INTRODUCTION

Building a strong, team-oriented atmosphere in your salon is a never-ending task. It must begin with good hiring skills and be followed by a continuing training program. This shows your ability as a strong leader as well as a motivator of your staff.

One of the most important factors in building a team is to listen to your staff members. When you listen, they realize you consider them part of the future of the salon and its success. Always be willing to listen to your staff, whether they are offering creative promotional ideas, discussing technical issues, or presenting the occasional unwanted gripe. Look at the unwanted gripe as an opportunity instead of a negative situation. If staff members are willing to voice their gripes to you, they are saying, "I really like working for you, but..." They are giving you the opportunity to solve what could later become a larger problem or a walk-out.

When the doors to communication are open to your team and their creativity is accepted with genuine appreciation, they will no doubt come up with ideas that might never occur to you. These ideas could lead to exciting ways to achieve a much healthier bottom line.

❧ DEVELOPING A TEAM CONCEPT

The following ideas will help you establish a united salon workforce:

- ❧ Establish salon standards that reflect your ideas, goals, and your salon's personality.
- ❧ Develop a business plan.
- ❧ Develop a salon policy and procedures manual.
- ❧ Hold staff meetings on a regular basis. Do not hold gripe sessions. These meetings should be positive and motivating.
- ❧ At meetings, stress the importance of working together for the good of the salon as a whole and each other as a team.
- ❧ Always set good examples. Your staff will react to your actions.
- ❧ Make your staff aware at all times that they are important to you and the success of your salon.
- ❧ When you make a mistake—and you will—be willing to admit it and discuss ways of correcting the mistake.
- ❧ Always expect the best of your staff and yourself.
- ❧ Be loyal to your staff. You can expect loyalty only when you give loyalty.

The following characteristics will help you determine if you have a united team of employees:

Recognizing Your Team

- ❧ Everyone knows he or she can ask for help from someone else in the salon at any time and get it.

Even the so-called salon hot shots, or stars, are willing to do the towels, brushes, and other dreaded chores.

- ❧ The client always comes first.
- ❧ Clients feel free to try new or different stylists.
- ❧ During staff meetings, stylists feel free to speak up with ideas or problems.

- Staff members know they are treated as an important part of the salon.

You Know You Have Lost Your Team When...

- Certain staff members feel they don't have to help with the so-called menial tasks.
- Clients go to another salon when their stylist isn't available.
- There is a lack of interest or indifference during staff meetings.
- Clients notice tension among certain staff members.
- Staff members repeatedly miss meetings or educational events for the advancement of their education.
- You constantly hear "It's not MY job."

Try the tips presented throughout the rest of this chapter to build unity among your employees.

Fifty Ways to Keep Your Employees Happy

1. Create a service-oriented culture.
   - All employees must be service oriented.
   - Service-oriented employees are loyalty oriented.
2. Have a service vision.
   - When employees see a vision, they feel directed.
   - Your staff feels a sense of importance in carrying out your vision.
3. Offer total support.
   - By offering support, you are showing you care.
   - You should always be supportive of employee growth.
   - Offer support, even when an employee decides to leave. (He or she may decide to come back.)
4. Put your policies in writing.
   - This is very important to your staff so they know what you expect.

- Unwritten expectations are never achieved.
- Your staff deserves to have advance knowledge of procedures.

5. Encourage employee empowerment.
   - Give your staff the authority to make decisions regarding the servicing of clients.
   - Allow your staff to make joint decisions that affect them in a positive nature.

6. Offer ongoing employee training.
   - By offering training, you are investing in your staff.
   - You are sending a message that you value them.
   - You will reap the benefits of educated staff.

7. Market your service program.
   - Market to the clientele you want to reach.
   - Your staff should reap the benefits of marketing of their attributes.

8. Hire the right people.
   - Take *time* to hire the right people.
   - Hire customer-oriented people.
   - Hire team players.

9. Don't forget the little things.
   - Pleasant surprises are a real delight.
   - Offer open recognition of employee achievements.
   - Offer creative perks (This may include payroll savings plans or providing lunch or continental breakfast one day a week.)

10. Reward loyalty.
    - What gets rewarded gets repeated.
    - Reward both clients and employees.
    - Offer rewards with perceived value (not necessarily expensive rewards).

11. Inspect what you expect.
    - If you have performance or quota expectations, follow the progress of employees.
    - Everyone must know how you judge performance.
12. Set standards of performance.
    - Set standards for the salon, thus establishing criteria for employee behavior and operational procedures.
    - Set standards for the salon image.
    - Set standards for the quality of service.
13. Allow and encourage movement.
    - Encourage staff to move their stations.
    - Encourage interaction among staff and employees.
14. Cross train.
    - Encourage staff to be proficient in many areas of salon services. This helps prevent burnout.
15. Establish user-friendly service.
    - Train staff to be aware of clients' needs and to be available to the client.
    - Be aware of your staff's needs.
16. Allow for flexibility in your salon policies.
    - Rigid is as rigid does (Too tight control often leads to a rebellious environment caused by a lack of willingness to negotiate.)
    - Rules are made to be broken.
    - Flexibility breeds creativity.
17. Educate your employees to educate your clients.
    - Your staff should learn to educate the client on the service being performed as well as the products used.
    - Bring someone in (e.g., a vendor, an instructor from a beauty school) to educate staff members on the latest, newest techniques.

18. Handle complaints properly.
    - Don't let a molehill become a mountain.
    - When an employee complains, that is a good sign.
    - When employees don't complain, worry—communication has broken down.
19. Turn complaints into opportunities.
    - When an employee complains, you have the opportunity to make positive changes for everyone.
    - When you address a complaint in a positive way, you are saying "I care."
20. Train employees to do the job right the first time.
    - Encourage staff to take their time with the client, to listen and understand what the client is asking for.
    - Less redo's means more money for the stylist, which translates into a happier stylist.
21. Remember, each employee is a potential lifetime investment.
    - Spend time and money on developing a valuable employee.
    - The cost of replacing a lost employee is astronomical compared to the cost of simply keeping the employee satisfied.
22. Ask for staff feedback.
    - Don't be afraid to implement staff members' ideas.
    - Your staff should feel comfortable making suggestions to you.
23. Identify your staff's needs.
    - Do they need to sell retail?
    - Do they need to sell services?
    - Do they need to promote business?
    - They all need to feel wanted and valued.
24. Ask for and use staff ideas.
    - When you ask, be sure to utilize responses.
    - If you ask and then ignore, you are sending a negative statement.

25. Be fair and consistent.
    - Your staff deserves to know what to expect from you at all times.
    - Staff should never have to wonder what kind of mood are you are in.
    - Discipline should always be the same for everyone.
    - If something was wrong yesterday, it is wrong today.
26. Underpromise and overdeliver.
    - When hiring, only promise what you can deliver.
    - Don't promise the moon on a cloudy night.
27. Compete on benefits, not higher commissions.
    - Offer better working conditions.
    - Offer a better benefit package.
    - Offer better products.
    - Never try to match other salons' higher commission rates. (Too often, salon owners feel compelled to pay higher commissions than they can afford simply because they feel pressured to compete.)
28. High touch is more important than high tech.
    - A caring salon offers much more security than a high-tech salon.
    - Working conditions are extremely important to all employees.
    - A feeling of caring will retain an employee far more than the latest equipment.
29. Ask staff members what they want.
    - When you ask what your staff wants, you show you care.
    - Don't assume you know what they want.
30. Maintain daily service management.
    - Be aware of your salon's condition at all times.
    - Be aware of the service being offered to clients.
    - Be aware of the service you are providing to your staff.

31. Realize the cost of a lost employee.
    - When you lose an employee, you risk salon morale.
    - When you lose an employee, you lose clients and income.
    - When you lose an employee, you must replace him or her (at great expense).
    - When you lose an employee, you must replace lost clients.
32. Know your competition.
    - Make every effort to know how the competition hires, trains, offers benefits, and compensates employees.
    - By keeping up with the compensation, you can offset any potential problems with staff expecting what cannot be delivered.
33. Conduct market research on a regular basis.
    - Know what the local market can bear in costs.
    - Know what services to promote and whom to promote to.
34. Conduct internal assessments.
    - Work with your staff to conduct assessments of your existing clients.
    - Conduct assessments of your employees in which they provide their input about the services being offered, the products customers want, etc.
35. Know what your staff members need, want, and expect.
    - Don't be afraid to question your staff.
    - When you need to make changes, do so.
36. Find, nurture, and acknowledge salon champions.
    - When you have superstars, acknowledge them
    - Give plaques, ribbons, etc.
    - If you've got stars, flaunt them!
37. Remember, effective communication is critical to success.
    - Learn to communicate honestly with your staff.
    - Listening is an art that should be practiced often.

38. Rapport is the key to successful communication.

    ❧ Rapport is developed through trust.

    ❧ Trust is built by delivering what is promised.

    ❧ Caring about the well-being of your staff, leads to trust and the foundation of a long-lasting relationship.

39. Smile.

    ❧ When all else fails, a smile will see you through anything.

    ❧ No words are needed when a smile is present.

40. Make employees feel important.

    ❧ Don't hesitate to praise when it is appropriate.

    ❧ Always look for the opportunity to offer words of encouragement.

    ❧ Always look for the good in everyone.

41. Promote your employees.

    ❧ Most local newspapers have business briefs or features that are available for announcing employee accomplishments. These are usually free of charge.

    ❧ By promoting your employees' accomplishments, you are promoting your salon and the fact that you care about your employees' future.

    ❧ Encourage your employees to take part in local community events.

42. Create an employee council.

    ❧ Develop a team within your salon to come up with ideas to enhance the working conditions in the salon, the promotion of the salon, and any other issues relating to the salon's environment.

    ❧ Find a way to implement the suggestions of your council.

43. Develop a power point system.

    ❧ Implement a reward system for your employees.

    ❧ Offer points for milestones reached.

    ❧ Always have a goal that your employees are striving to reach. Be sure the reward justifies the accomplishment.

44. Accept only excellence.

- ✿ You set the standards for your salon, and everyone in your employ should be able to live up to those standards.

- ✿ Set standards that are achievable.

45. Remember, employees are clients, too.

- ✿ Treat your employees with the same courtesy that you would a client.

- ✿ Place a high value on your employees, and strive to retain them.

46. Show employees you care.

- ✿ This can't be stressed enough. If you don't show you care, someone else will.

- ✿ Employees often leave due to lack of respect and caring.

47. Display employee accomplishments.

- ✿ Have an employee wall where you display the employee plaques, certificates, etc.

- ✿ Start an employee brag book. Keep it in the reception area. Show off your staff's talents.

48. Go the extra mile.

- ✿ If you go the extra mile, your staff will not be going down the block for an additional 5% commission.

- ✿ Little things mean everything.

49. Expect professionalism.

- ✿ Professionalism breeds professionals.

50. Remember, employees react to our actions.

- ✿ The days of "do as I say, not as I do" are long gone. You cannot expect your employees to act one way if you are acting another.

- ✿ If you exhibit pride in working in your salon, your staff will be proud to be there as well.

Chapter 7

Employees versus Booth Rental and Contractors

 INTRODUCTION

The hiring of employees versus the use of booth rental and contractors is probably one of the most controversial issues facing the salon industry today. There is no perfect system that works for everyone. The important factor is to choose a system that is satisfactory to you and your staff—a system that will allow for a healthy profit margin for your salon.

This chapter provides enough information to enable you to decide to rent a booth, be an independent contractor or open a booth rental or independent contractor salon, or remain employee based. Your decision should be based on your particular needs and your career goals. It should also be based on legal factors. You must know all of the rules that govern the way you work or run your business.

All states are different and have regulations that are geared only for that state. However, the federal guidelines are the same throughout the entire country. In this chapter, many of the rules and regulations have been compiled. If I have failed to address an issue you have concerns about, feel free to contact our office and we will do our best to answer your questions.

The information presented in this chapter is accurate and current to the best of our knowledge. We have gone to the most reliable sources for confirmation and updated information. However, rules do change rapidly, and we cannot take responsibility for the operation of your personal situation or your salon. Many of the Internal Revenue Service (IRS) rules and regulations are subject to the interpretation of the individual auditor. Therefore, we must add a disclaimer that National Alliance of Salon Professionals cannot take responsibilities for your actions as a booth renter, independent contractor, or salon owner with booth renters or independent contractors.

The contracts provided in the Appendix of this book are to be used only as guidelines for your particular situation and should not be used as is without first consulting your accountant and/or your tax attorney.

THE IRS AND YOU

For years, we have been hearing, "The IRS is coming! The IRS is coming!" The truth is, the IRS is already here, and IRS auditors know that booth renters are here. Contrary to what many in the beauty industry may want to believe, the two can co-habituate. The IRS requires that you, as a citizen of the United States, pay tax. If your employer is not withholding taxes for you, then you must pay taxes directly to the IRS. The bottom line is, someone is responsible for income tax being paid. I don't think the IRS really cares who it is. But you can bet they will come looking to someone for the tax if it is not paid.

No matter how you choose to operate as a beauty professional, it is important that you do it legally and professionally. Now let's move on to the criteria that govern how you operate.

The following Compliance Checklist is a simple test to find out how much you already know about contracting regulations. The Appendix of this book contains another copy of the test, which you can use to determine if you fully understand all the implications of the information presented in this chapter.

Compliance Checklist

Carefully study the issues listed below and place a checkmark under the party you feel is responsible for each. If you are a contractor at this time, consider the way you are operating now and use that as your guide.

ISSUE	NOT APPLICABLE	SALON OWNER	CONTRACTOR
Telephone			
Cash Register			
Monies			
Retail Product			
Liability Insurance			
Business Cards			
Marketing Customers			
Promotions			
Receptionist			
Appointment Book			
Back Bar Supplies			
Station Supplies			
Chemical Products			
Small Equipment			
Large Equipment			
Sundry Products (cotton, etc.)			
Cleaning (booth/sink area, etc.)			
Cleaning Common Area (reception, bathroom, etc.)			
Meetings			
W-2 Forms			
1099 Forms			
Hiring Assistants			
Training and Advance Education			
Occupational License			

EMPLOYING VERSUS RENTING AND CONTRACTING

There are many factors to consider before renting a booth or acting as an independent contractor. Let's establish a basic understanding of each.

Employees

Generally, employees can be defined either under common law or under statutes for special purposes.

COMMON LAW EMPLOYEES

Anyone who performs a service that can be controlled by an employer (what will be done and how it will be done) is an employee. This is so even when the employer has the legal right to control the method and results of the service.

Generally, people in business for themselves are not employees. For example, doctors, lawyers, construction contractors, and others in an independent trade in which they offer their services to the public, such as hairstylists and barbers, could be considered nonemployees.

If an employer/employee relationship exists, it does not matter what it is called. The employee may be called a partner, agent, or independent contractor. It also does not matter how payments are measured or paid, what they are called, or whether the employee works full or part time.

Whether an employer/employee relationship exists will be determined by guidelines under Section 312(d) of the Internal Revenue Code of 1986 and by long-standing common law tests. Publication 937, Employment Taxes, gives an example of the employer/employee relationship.

If you want the IRS to decide whether a worker is an employee, file form SS-8, Information for Use in Determining Whether a Worker is an Employee for Purposes of Federal Employment Taxes and Income Tax Withholding. The form is available at IRS offices. You will find a sample of the SS-8 form in the Appendix of this book.

Independent Contractors

The independent contractor (IC) is not the same as a booth renter. However, in many states ICs are considered the same for the purpose of collecting sales tax. The independent contractor usually pays the salon owner a percentage of his or her income for each given week. Some other guidelines are as follows:

- The independent contractor must handle his or her own monies.
- The salon owner usually is paid a percentage of the IC's income.
- The IC must pay sales tax on the monies paid to the salon owner.
- Taxes are paid by the IC.
- The IC has a key to the salon and can come and go as he or she pleases.

The IRS usually frowns on this type of relationship because it is extremely hard to adhere to all of the imposed guidelines. The IRS likes things to be cut and dry in nature. For that reason it is far better to enter into a rental situation if you are not going to operate as an employee or employer.

Booth Renters

Booth renters simply pay a set amount of rent to the salon owner each week. This is an established amount of rent that is the same every week and does not vary according to the amount of work the renter does. This method is by far the safest way to operate, other than employee based. The salon owner must realize that there can be absolutely no control exercised over the booth renter. The salon owner in this case is merely a landlord. The booth renter must pay sales tax on the amount of rent.

The actual rules governing booth renters are the same as for independent contractors. The IRS is much more favorable to rental situations as opposed to contractor status. Other factors to consider are as follows:

- There is complete separation between the owner and the renter.
- Contracts spell out everything.
- The salon owner has no control over the renter.
- The salon owner cannot supply products, insurance, etc.

PROCEDURES REGARDING INDEPEN-DENT CONTRACTORS AND RENTERS

The contractor or renter must provide the salon owner/landlord with a form 1099 at the end of the year. In addition, there are two overriding points that must always be maintained in a salon owner/independent relationship:

1. Separation of relationship—there is no employee/ employer relationship.
2. The IC must have complete control of the operation of his or her business.

For renters and ICs, there are three predominant issues that a government agency looks at during a status classification audit:

1. Is there a contract that clearly describes a landlord/tenant relationship in all aspects?
2. There must be a flat rate of rent clearly specified in the contract, and it must be kept completely separate from any other monies or fees collected.
3. The salon owner or landlord is not allowed to handle or control the actual monies received for services rendered by the

Renters will be responsible for Liability Insurance and on personal possessor

Renters will enter this agreement on ___ paying the first wks rent + the ___

IC in any form or fashion. All checks written out by the clients for services received must be made out to the IC.

Salon owners must look at themselves as landlords and at all of the individual renters as individual stores or businesses.

Although the lease must have a flat rate of rent included, it can include opportunities for added income. The following are some of the possibilities for added income. These must be considered carefully and thoroughly researched and planned for your particular situation.

1. The landlord is allowed to own a separate retail center in the salon while disallowing the IC to sell his or her own retail products. The landlord can pay a commission to the IC for any retail the IC is responsible for selling. This will be paid in a check separate from anything else. The IC will receive a form 1099 from the salon owner at the end of the year reflecting the monies received during the year from retail sales.

2. The landlord/salon owner can provide the use of a charge card machine (Mastercard and Visa) to the IC for an additional fee based on a percentage of the actual sale.

3. The landlord/salon owner can provide a receptionist service for an additional fee. This could include answering the phone and scheduling appointments. Should the IC choose not to subscribe to this service, a phone system should be in place with separate.lines for each station. The phone system would be programmable either to be answered at the central desk or to go directly to the individual station. ICs can choose to put in their own separate line directly at their own station.

4. The option to receive new customers generated by salon-initiated advertising is also a service that can be provided. The IC can be charged a one-time fee for the nonrequest client as an advertising or finder's fee.

The key to these additional services is that the IC is given the choice to accept or decline the use of any or all of the optional services provided by the landlord/salon owner. The fees paid for these services must be kept separate in payment and structure from the flat rate rent payment. The IC must provide separate checks for these services.

The landlord/salon owner must have the right to sublease the space within the salon if it is being leased by the landlord/salon owner from another source (not owned by the landlord/salon owner).

There must be a lease between the salon owner and the independent contractor/booth renter to indicate that an independent contractor/booth renter situation exists. The lease should spell out the exact manner in which the relationship will be carried out. It is also advisable to file an SS-8 form with the IRS. This form determines the eligibility of the salon to operate as an independent contractor salon.

ARTICLES OF SEPARATION

The IRS looks for total separation when making their decisions about the eligibility of a salon for IC status. The IRS looks for separation in the following areas:

Taxes

- Contractor/renter pays all of his or her own federal, state, and local taxes.
- Contractor/renter must have and show proof of all business licenses,. including state, county, and city.
- Contractor/renter must have his or her own sales tax number for product sales.
- The landlord/salon owner should prorate the sales tax received against those they are required to pay on their salon rent.

Contract

- There must be a contract between the landlord/salon owner and the contractor/renter. It must be specific and precise.
- The SS-8 form should be filed by both the landlord/salon owner and the contractor/renter.

Advertising and Marketing

- Business cards should be the sole responsibility of the contractor/renter.
- If the salon furnishes the cards, the contractor/renter's name should be at least as large as the salon's name.
- Contractor/renter should do his or her own advertising (yellow pages, newspaper, promotions, etc.)
- The salon can only advertise for contractors/renters if they are being paid a fee for the service.

Insurance

- Contractor/renter is responsible for his or her own liability and malpractice insurance and should be required to show landlord/salon owner proof of coverage in order to rent space.

Retail Sales

- Contractor/renter can not sell his or her own products in his or her individual area.
- Landlord/salon owner can provide retail products and pay contractor/renter commission (landlord/salon owner must give contractor/renter a form 1099 reflecting commission paid).

General Salon Operation

- Landlord/salon owner must have legal rights to sublease space.
- Sales tax must be collected for space rent and sent in to Department of Revenue. (Check with your state to see if this is a requirement for you.)
- Appointments must be made by contractors/renters.
- IRS prefers that contractors/renters have their own phone.
- Monies cannot be handled by landlord/salon owner or their receptionist unless a fee is paid for such service.
- Monies cannot be placed in the bank account of the landlord/contractor.
- Landlord/salon owner cannot give regular paychecks to contractor/renter.
- Products for use at stations or back bar cannot be furnished by landlord/salon owner.
- Landlord/salon owner cannot call mandatory meetings unless pertaining to the lease or state-regulated or legal issues.

In the Appendix of this book, you will find two contracts for your use as guides only. These will give you an idea of what you should consider putting in your own contract, or what to expect if you are an independent contractor/renter. These are not to be used as is. Modify them with the help of your attorney or certified public accountant.

The following list is the Internal Revenue Service 20 Rules test for eligibility.[1] There are many items that could be considered gray areas, especially if you are an independent contractor as opposed to a booth renter. Follow these rules to the letter. If you have questions about them, contact our office and we will try to clarify them for you. We can be reached by phone at (904) 385-7668 or by mail at P.O. Box 4307, Tallahassee, Florida 32315.

---

[1] A copy of the IRS 20 Rules test can be obtained at a local IRS office. They are listed in the IRS Employment Taxes Publication #937.

1. *Instructions*: A worker who is required to comply with another person's instructions about when, where, and how to work is ordinarily an employee. The salon owner cannot give any help in the operation of the contractor's work.

2. *Training*: Training a worker indicates that the employer exercises control over the means by which the result is accomplished. The salon owner cannot take the initiative in training the contractor at all. Salon owners can, however, offer classes and invite the contractors to come as guests or at a charge. This cannot be a mandatory workshop.

3. *Integration*: When the success or continuation of a business depends on the performance of certain services, the worker performing those services is subject to a certain amount of control by the owner of the business. This simply means that the salon owner cannot let the performance of the contractor's business determine the success of his or her own business.

4. *Services rendered personally*: If the services must be rendered personally, the employer controls both the means and the results of the work. Unless stipulated otherwise in the contract, the contractor has the right to hire or sublet his or her space if not able to be at work or on vacation. This should always be covered in the contract.

5. *Hiring, supervising, and paying assistants:* Control is exercised if the employer hires, supervises, and pays assistants. The contractors have the right to hire their own assistants or, when applicable, use assistants hired by the salon owner if they paid a fee for the service of the assistants.

6. *Continuing relationship:* A continuing relationship between the worker and the employer indicates that an employer/employee relationship exists. The IRS views a continuing relationship as one in which the salon owner pays for services rendered and the contractor takes his or her monies and leaves. Any yearly payments over $10,000 are considered a continuing relationship.

7. *Set hours of work:* The establishment of set hours of work by

the employer indicates control. The contractor must be free to work the hours of his or her choice.

8. *Full time required:* If the worker must devote full time to the employer's business, the employer has control over the worker's time. An independent contractor is free to work when and for whom he or she chooses.

9. *Doing work on the employer's premises:* Control is indicated if the work is performed on the employer's premises. Again, this relates to the IRS assumption that contractors do the work and leave.

10. *Order or sequence set:* Control is indicated if a worker is not free to choose his or her own pattern of work, but must perform services in the sequence set by the employer. The results of the contractor's work cannot depend on the assistance or guidance of the salon owner.

11. *Oral or written reports:* Control is indicated if the worker must submit regular oral or written reports to the employer. The contractor cannot be required to give reports of income to the salon owner. In a percentage-based contract, this would be necessary and, under most situations, not legal.

12. *Payment by hour, week, or month:* Payment by the hour, week, or month points to an employer/employee relationship. An independent contractor is usually paid by the job. The salon owner should not be paying the contractor a paycheck on a regular basis, and especially no more than $10,000 per year.

13. *Payment of business expenses:* Payment of the worker's business and/or traveling expenses is indicative of an employer/employee relationship. This is not allowed for any reason. If the salon owner takes responsibility for the business expenses of the contractor, that definitely shows control.

14. *Tools and supplies:* If the employer furnishes significant tools or supplies necessary to the performance of the worker's job, then an employer/employee relationship exists. The salon owner is not allowed to supply back bar or station products. No products needed for the performance of the contractor's job can be furnished by the salon owner.

15. *Significant investment:* A worker is an independent contractor if he or she invests in facilities that are not typically maintained by employee. The contractor's investment in his or her business must be significant, showing ownership.

16. *Realization of profit or loss:* A worker who can realize a profit or loss is an independent contractor. The worker who cannot is generally an employee.

17. *Working for more than one firm at a time:* If a worker is free to work for more than one firm at a time, he or she is usually an independent contractor. The contractor has the right to work for as many different salons as he or she wishes.

18. *Making service available to the general public:* A worker is usually an independent contractor if he or she makes his or her services available to the general public on a regular and consistent basis. Again, the contractor can work for anyone he or she chooses at any time and any place.

19. *Right to discharge:* The right of the employer to discharge a worker indicates that he or she is an employee. You cannot fire or be fired in a contractor status. There must be a lease contract that states the way the working relationship will end.

20. *Right to terminate:* A worker is an employee if he or she has the right to end his or her relationship with his or her principal at any time he or she wishes without incurring liability. The contractor does not have the right to quit or leave. The same holds true here as in item 19. There must be a contract that states the way of ending the working relationship.

Chapter 8

Setting and Raising Prices

 ## INTRODUCTION

Raising prices is one of the hardest decisions that you will have to face. We all hate to do it. We are afraid of losing clients, which would counteract the revenue gain from the increase in price. Often, we feel it is necessary to raise prices, but we don't know how much is called for. We don't want to go too high, but if we don't raise the price enough, we will be faced with the same situation again in a few months or, worse, be stuck with prices that don't allow for a profit.

 ## FORMULA FOR PRICE SETTING

If you feel the time is right for a price increase, take the proper steps *now*. Your clients have chosen your salon for several reasons: location, prices, atmosphere, professionalism, quality of service, etc. Consider the following:

- If you have a reputation for high volume and low service, your fears of raising prices may be well founded. If you must make more money, consider increasing productivity and cutting your costs rather than increasing prices.
- If you have a low-volume, high-service salon, your clientele will not be greatly affected by a reasonable increase. You will most likely lose one or two clients, but they often return for the quality service they were accustomed to.

Compare your prices with similar salons in your area. Be sure to compare with salons that offer services similar to those of your salon. Problems resulting from increased prices are often not due to the increase itself, but to the manner in which the increase was presented.

Many salon owners have a tendency to put off raising prices, even after they have decided to do so, and even at the expense of risking the financial security of their salons. Perhaps their stylists intimidate them with fears that the stylists' clients won't pay higher prices. Perhaps the salon owners feel that the salon's clients won't stand for the increase. Perhaps there is a new "cheapy" salon just around the corner from the salon and thus the change should not be made immediately Whatever the reason may be, it is important that you first make sure you feel justified in making the changes. It is a known fact that the beauty industry has not kept up with the rising rate of inflation. The national rate of profit in this industry is a little above 6%. Even this minor amount of profit is reached by only the most budget-minded salon owners.

Careful planning will make the price increase painless and profitable. Make your staff aware of the necessity for the price increase. Hold a staff meeting before your increase and explain the procedure in detail. When staff members understand your need, they will be likely to give you their support. Keep in mind the following suggestions:

- Don't make the price change face to face. Send out newsletters at least six weeks in advance of the projected increase date. Include a salon menu giving prices of all services performed in your salon. The client has the right to know prices before committing to the service.
- Have your receptionist be the one who handles all money transactions. This eliminates the stylists charging different prices.
- Display an attractive printed price list. Post the list in your reception area. Again, clients want to be aware of costs.
- Give your clients more for their money. Extra services don't cost you anything. Offer that extra care so cherished by the client. A little attention goes a long way in retaining clients.

Remind yourself that you want to make a profit. You cannot justify the time, stress, and headaches of owning your own business if all you accomplish is making ends meet. Your salary is *not* part of your profit. Your salon profit is figured after you deduct your salary and all of the other expenses.

FORMULA FOR UNDERSTANDING SERVICE INCOME

The following information will help you see the potential for profits on the services your staff performs. Use this as a tool to understand the costs you are responsible for on services done in your salon. Our example is based on $500 in services with 55% commission paid.

Weekly Gross Pay	$275.00
Costs Per Week	
Paid Vacation	
$275 / 52 weeks	$5.29
Paid Holidays (3 days per year)	
3 days x 8 hours per day = 24 hours per year	
24 hours x $6.87 per hour = $164.88 per year	
$164.88 per year / 52 weeks =	$3.17
Insurance ($60 per month)	
$60 per month x 12 months = $720 per year	
$720 per year / 52 weeks =	$13.85
Education	
$100 per year / 52 weeks =	$1.92
TOTAL: Weekly Gross Pay including benefits =	**$299.23**
TOTAL: Adjusted Hourly Costs =	**$ 7.48**

Social Security per week	
Gross pay + taxable benefits	
(vacation, holidays) =	$283.46
$283.46 x 7.65% social security =	$21.68
Subtotal: Gross pay + Social Security +	
nontaxable benefits (insur., educ.)	**$320.91**
Worker's Compensation	
1.36% x $320.91 =	$4.36
State Unemployment	
1% x $320.91 =	$.32
Federal Unemployment	
2.7% x $320.91 =	$8.66
TOTAL: Labor Costs =	**$334.25**
TOTAL: Adjusted Hourly Costs =	**$ 8.36**

Out of every $500 in services your salon performs, the stylist receives $334.25. The salon will actually keep only $165.75. This is before salon expenses such as rent, utilities, supplies, and all other expenses. Use this scale as a tool to find ways of increasing your profits. You must be aware of costs.

KNOW YOUR PROFIT SERVICES

It is important to know which services you make a profit on and which you lose money on. There is a simple calculation for determining where your money is made. First, determine your costs. These include fixed costs, product costs, and labor. Fixed costs (overhead) include rent, utilities, advertising, office supplies, benefits, etc. As an example, let's use $50,000 as our per year fixed costs.

- A salon is open 50 hours per week, 50 weeks per year, or 2500 hours per year.
- It has four styling chairs, multiplied by the 2500 hours per year. This allows for 10,000 chair hours available for clients.
- Divide the fixed costs ($50,000) by the chair hours (10,000), and the fixed cost per chair hour is $5.

It is not realistic to expect 100% total booked hours. We are going to use 75% booked hours for our example. This gives us 7500 booked chair hours and a fixed cost of $6.67.

Product costs include perms, colors, etc. We will use perms as our example. We also include cotton coil, shampoo, end papers, etc., to be approximately $5.

Labor costs include all money paid to the stylist, which we figured at 55%.

Example 1: $1^1/_2$- hour perm service

$\quad$ $ 45.00 per price

$\quad$ − 5.00 product price

$\quad$ − 6.67 fixed costs

$\quad$ − 24.75 labor (55% commission)

$\quad$ $ 8.58 profit (approx. 19%)

This is a fairly good profit margin. Keep in mind that the product costs for each service will vary greatly and affect your profit/loss margins. Let's look at the average shampoo and set.

Example 2: $1/2$-hour shampoo/set service

$ 10.00 $1/2$-hour shampoo set service
  −   .75 product costs
  −   3.34 fixed costs ($1/2$ hour)
  −   5.50 labor (55% commission)
$ .41 profit (approx. 4%)

As you can see, there is a big difference between the profit generated from one service and that from another. It is important to take advantage of this knowledge and learn to make profitable services more profitable and less profitable services more profitable. If you know which services generate the least profit, you'll be better able to make the necessary adjustments. Should you cut costs? Can you shorten the amount of time needed to perform the service? Should you raise your price? These are questions to consider.

▓ PAY YOURSELF FIRST

Often, in the beauty industry, salon owners leave fate to decide the amount of profit realized. More often than not, the profit margin is less than 10%. Why not sit down with your true salon figures and decide how much of a profit you want to have at the end of each month and work it into your price structure? The following formula will guarantee a profit.

If you know that your operating expenses (rent, advertising, utilities, telephone, etc.) are $4200 a month and you want to make a profit of $2000 a month, you have total costs to offset $6200 a month: $4200 (operating costs) + $2000 (desired profit) = $6200. The $6200 is the amount of gross profit you need to generate. Gross profit is what's left after you've paid all the costs directly associated with creating sales, like payroll costs, buying products, etc.

The next step is to determine how much your labor and product costs are for every dollar in sales. In the beauty industry, labor and product costs run between $.45 and $.75 per $1 in sales. The biggest portion of this amount is usually commission. If you pay your staff 50% commission or more, you will be toward the high range ($.65 to $.70). If you are making good product purchases and controlling your inventory, you might be able to get that figure down to $.50 to $.55. For example, let's use $.60 as our total labor and product costs. If $.60 (or 60%) of every dollar the salon takes in is used to pay for labor and products, then $.40 is left over to pay for operating expenses and profit. Your gross profit margin is 40%.

The next step is estimating total sales. You take your total profits and overhead costs of $6200 and divide it by the 40% gross profit margin: $6200 (operating expense + profit) + .40 (gross profit margin) = $15,500. In this example, you would need $15,500 in total monthly sales to break even. But you didn't just break even, you had built in $2000 in profits. This is just another way of paying yourself first.

You want to make sure that you have a firm control of operating expenses. However, you might overspend on an item such as advertising. If you choose to spend an extra $300, you must add that to the $4200 from our example. What does that do to your break-even figure? You still want the profits of $2000, so you add the $300 to the $6200 you've allocated to operating expenses and profits. You now have $6500. Divide that by your 40% and you come up with $16,250. While you have increased your operating expenses by only $300, you've had to increase sales by $750 just to pay for the additional $300.

On the other hand, what happens if your 40% gross profit margin changes? In other words, you might not be taking advantage of volume discounts, you might be overstocked, or maybe you have more receptionist hours than you expected. Your product and labor costs would go up; instead of paying $.60 for your product and labor costs, maybe you would pay $.65. If you are still trying to maintain the $4200 in operating costs and the $2000 in profits, $.65 in labor and product costs would cause your gross profit margin to decrease to 35% and your break-even figure to move up to $17,714.

As you can see, the most critical issue is that only five percentage points in labor and product costs drive your break-even point much higher — $2214 higher. This is why building profits into your salon goals aids you in maintaining a margin for error. If you have some unexpected expense, you have a budgeted cushion for meeting those needs. Of course, if you don't have any unusual expenses and you make your projections, you have $2000 in profit to use as you want. And that is your main objective.

SHOULD YOU COMPUTERIZE?

Most successful managers make good decisions based on good information about their business: what's profitable and what isn't; what is productive and what (or who) isn't; what's working and what isn't. For most businesses, information is not just vital but expensive. Before computers, the salon owner who wanted reliable information about the salon's operation had to spend long, tedious hours going over receipts, client cards, and appointment books. This took the owner away from other tasks that could have brought more money into the salon: advertising, marketing, mailing, client consulting, counseling with staff members, etc.

Now that information is available literally at the owner's fingertips, quickly, and inexpensively. As an owner, you know that the computer won't make any decisions for you, but it will give you all the information you need to make the best decisions for your salon. Automating your salon could well be one of the best decisions you will ever make. Computers make your business more, not less, personal. You can use your computer to personalize your client mailings. You can use it to keep track of individual preferences. You'll find that the number of repeat visits goes up and you lose fewer clients because your mailings now have a personal touch.

By saving time, salon automation saves you money. With computers, payroll takes only minutes, and inventory is always exact. Other benefits include the following:

- You have accurate, up-to-the-minute financial reports; you and your accountant spend less time figuring out your finances.
- You can see your budget at a glance and know exactly where you stand.
- You can automate your cash drawer to reduce errors and control theft.
- You can record all point-of-sale transactions instantly.
- The computer handles payroll; it computes a paycheck in seconds, even with the most complex compensation system. Commissions and deductions are automatically figured and clearly shown.
- Accounts payable are clearly recorded and tracked.
- Your computerized appointment book is neat, clear, accessible, quick, and easily corrected.
- The computer tracks services: percent of growth or decline, which ones are stagnating and need promotion.
- The computer handles product inventory: automatic ordering, overstocking, loss control; you'll spend less time on your retail inventory and know so much more about your retail business.
- The computer provides individualized product prescriptions automatically to stimulate retail sales.
- The computer tracks staff performance and total sales.
- The computer tracks services sales by category, average service sales per client, etc.
- The computer tracks retail sales per product, average sales per client.

- The computer records the average ticket per client.
- The computer tracks your salon's productivity—the dollars brought in per hour.
- The computer keeps track of client base information.
- The computer generates reminders for clients that they are due for services.
- Client records are printed out automatically so your staff members know which products and services the client needs.
- The computer handles mailing lists; printing mailing labels is a snap. The mailings generated pertain to service reminders, promotions, special wishes for birthdays and anniversaries, etc.
- If one of your stylists quits, the computer can generate a letter immediately, enticing clients to remain with your salon.
- A newsletter is quick and easy to do on a computer.
- The computer tracks your advertising to see which ads draw customers. You can thus spend your money where it counts by dropping unproductive ads or promotions.
- The computer protects your client files by keeping them inaccessible except to authorized people using a password.

Every day that you operate without a computer is a day that you have spent time not making money. An exciting addition to owning a computer is to organize a computer user group and learn much, much more about the capabilities of computerization in the salon industry.

Appendix

CONTENTS

FORMULA FOR SERVICE INCOME

$____ in Services x____% Commmission = $____ weekly gross pay

$____ weekly gross pay / 40 hours per week = $____ hourly pay

---

Weekly Gross Pay $_____

Costs Per Week
Paid Vacation
     $_____ / 52 weeks $_____

Paid Holidays (3 days per year)
     3 days x 8 hours per day = 24 hours per year
     24 hours x $____ per hour = $____ per year
     $____ per year / 52 weeks = $_____

Insurance ($____ per month)
     $____ per month x 12 months = $____ per year
     $____ per year / 52 weeks = $_____

Education
     $____ per year / 52 weeks = $_____

TOTAL: Weekly Gross Pay including benefits = $_____
TOTAL: Adjusted Hourly Costs = $_____

Social Security per week
     Gross pay + taxable benefits
       (vacation, holidays) = $_____
     $____ x 7.65% social security = $_____

**Subtotal: Gross pay + Social Security +
nontaxable benefits (insur., educ.)** $_____

Worker's Compensation
     1.36% x $____ = $_____

State Unemployment
     1% x $____ = $_____

Federal Unemployment
     2.7% x $____ = $_____

TOTAL: Labor Costs = $_____
TOTAL: Adjusted Hourly Costs = $_____

Formula for Profits Services

Fixed expenses $_____

(a) Rent, utilities, cleaning, education
    insurance, professional services,
    advertisement, etc.   _____

Hours open per week   _____

Hours open per year   _____

Total hours available per year   _____

_____ Chairs x _____ available hours = _____ available chair hours

Fixed expense divided by chair hours = per hour overhead

    50% productivity = $_____ per hour overhead cost

    75% productivity = $_____ per hour overhead cost

55% Productivity

1$^1/_2$-hour perm service

$_____ perm price

$_____ product price

$_____ overhead cost

$_____ labor (@ 55% commission)

_____

$_____ profit (_____%)

55% Productivity

$^1/_2$-hour shampoo set service

$_____ product costs

$_____ fixed costs ($^1/_2$ hour)

$_____ labor (@ 55% commission)

_____

$_____ profit (_____%)

Government Forms: General Guidelines

1. Federal ID Number Application

   Application for a federal identification number is made on Form SS-, "Application for Employer Identification Number." When the Internal Revenue Service issues your number, they will also send you pertinent information about payroll tax withholdings and deposits, and payroll tax deposit coupons. If your business is a corporation, they will also send estimated income tax deposit coupons.

2. Employee's Withholding Allowance Certificate (W-4) and Employment Eligibility Verification (I-9)

   All new employees must fill out a Form W-4, "Employee Withholding Allowance Certificate," and an I-9, "Employment Eligibility Verification."

   The W-4 provides the employer with information necessary to withhold taxes from the employee's paycheck. It also provides the employee's Social Security number. This form should always be prepared before the employee begins work. There is a penalty for all W-2s filed annually with the Internal Revenue Service that don't have employee Social Security numbers.

   The I-9 is required by the Immigration and Naturalization Service and the Department of Labor. It is a method of verifying a person's citizenship status.

3. Wage and Tax Statement (W-2)

   By February 28 of each year, you are required to file a W-2, "Wage and Tax Statement," for each employee with the Internal Revenue Service and to furnish each employee with their copy. The employee copies of W-2s are to be distributed to employees by January 31 of each year.

   This form reports the total wages and withholding deducted for the previous calendar year. The total wages reported on each W-2 should equal the total taxable wages reported for the four quarterly 941 form. Income taxes withheld should agree with the quarterly 941s as well.

4. Employer's Annual Federal Unemployment (FUTA) Tax Return (940)

In addition to the quarterly state unemployment tax, there is a federal unemployment tax. Federal unemployment tax is reported on Form 940, "Employer's Annual Federal Unemployment Tax Report," and is due by January 31 of each year. This tax is computed at the rate of .008 (8/10 of 1%) for the first $7000 paid each employee each year (maximum of $56 per employee per year).

5. Employer's Quarterly Federal Tax Return (Form 940)

The deposit requirements for payment of taxes withheld from employees vary depending on the amount of liability. Most businesses and all new businesses fall into the category of having to make tax deposits monthly. Therefore, we will discuss the deposit requirements for monthly deposits. The IRS will notify employers each November if they are due to make deposits more frequently.

Computation of monthly tax liability:

Total FICA wages paid for the month	$ XXX.XX
Times .153	x .153
Total Social Security and Medicare tax liability	XXX.XX
Plus income taxes withheld	XXX.XX
Total tax liability for the month	$XXXX.XX

Each month the liability should be computed in this manner for tax withheld from wages *paid*. The emphasis is on *paid*, not *earned*. For example, the pay period for January would be included in February's computation and not January's.

By the 15th of each month, the tax liability for the previous month should be deposited in your commercial bank with a Federal Tax Deposit Coupon. Federal Tax Coupon Books will be mailed to you once a year by the Internal Revenue Service.

Each Coupon has two columns for identifying the type of tax being deposited and the tax period the deposit relates to. The type of tax should be identified by marking the box that corresponds with the tax form that the deposit relates. For example, for a deposit of FICA and income taxes, you would mark the box identified as 941 since the tax form filed with the IRS is just that—a form 941. You also must indicate the tax period to which the deposit relates. This is done by marking the appropriate quarter on the form. It is extremely important that you mark the correct quarter's box to make your deposit. Otherwise, the deposit will be credited to the wrong quarter and you will be overpaid in that quarter and underpaid in the quarter you intended to pay on and be penalized for under-payment of tax.

If the employer ever has a liability of over $100,000, a deposit is required by the next banking day.

6. U.S. Information Returns (Form 1099)

   Any person engaged in a trade or business who makes certain payments of $600 or more to an individual in the course of the trade or business must file an information return. If you pay dividends, interest, rents (not including real estate agents), fees, commissions, prizes, awards, or any other compensation for services rendered in the course of your trade or business to an individual who is not treated as an employee, you must furnish a 1099 annually to that person by January 31 of the following year. A copy must also be filed with the IRS by February 28.

7. Determination of Employee Work Status for Purposes of Federal Employment Taxes and Income Tax Withholding.

   This form should be filed by both the landlord/salon owner and the contractor/renter.

8. Employee's Report of Tips to Employer
   Another responsibility that falls on salon owners is the Tip Report. This is IRS form 4070, which can be obtained from your local IRS office. The cosmetologist is required to declare all tips on this form. Withholding and Social Security must be deducted from the tips received and you must match the social security. However, if the amount is less than $20, you are not required to do anything. Having the cosmetologist file this form each month frees you of any obligation. You must keep these forms in a file to back you in case of an audit.

Form **SS-4**
(Rev. December 1993)
Department of the Treasury
Internal Revenue Service

Application for Employer Identification Number

(For use by employers, corporations, partnerships, trusts, estates, churches, government agencies, certain individuals, and others. See instructions.)

EIN

OMB No. 1545-0003
Expires 12-31-96

Please type or print clearly.

1 Name of applicant (Legal name) (See instructions.)

2 Trade name of business, if different from name in line 1

3 Executor, trustee, "care of" name

4a Mailing address (street address) (room, apt., or suite no.)

5a Business address, if different from address in lines 4a and 4b

4b City, state, and ZIP code

5b City, state, and ZIP code

6 County and state where principal business is located

7 Name of principal officer, general partner, grantor, owner, or trustor—SSN required (See instructions.) ▶

8a Type of entity (Check only one box.) (See instructions.)
☐ Sole Proprietor (SSN) _____
☐ REMIC   ☐ Personal service corp.
☐ State/local government   ☐ National guard
☐ Other nonprofit organization (specify) _____
☐ Other (specify) ▶ _____

☐ Estate (SSN of decedent) _____
☐ Plan administrator-SSN _____
☐ Other corporation (specify) _____
☐ Federal government/military ☐ Church or church controlled organization
_____ (enter GEN if applicable) _____

☐ Trust
☐ Partnership
☐ Farmers' cooperative

8b If a corporation, name the state or foreign country (if applicable) where incorporated ▶

State

Foreign country

9 Reason for applying (Check only one box.)
☐ Started new business (specify) ▶ _____
☐ Hired employees
☐ Created a pension plan (specify type) ▶ _____
☐ Banking purpose (specify) ▶ _____

☐ Changed type of organization (specify) ▶ _____
☐ Purchased going business
☐ Created a trust (specify) ▶ _____
☐ Other (specify) ▶ _____

10 Date business started or acquired (Mo., day, year) (See instructions.)

11 Enter closing month of accounting year. (See instructions.)

12 First date wages or annuities were paid or will be paid (Mo., day, year). **Note:** *If applicant is a withholding agent, enter date income will first be paid to nonresident alien. (Mo., day, year)* . . . . ▶

13 Enter highest number of employees expected in the next 12 months. **Note:** *If the applicant does not expect to have any employees during the period, enter "0."* . . . . ▶

Nonagricultural	Agricultural	Household

14 Principal activity (See instructions.) ▶

15 Is the principal business activity manufacturing? . . . . ☐ Yes ☐ No
If "Yes," principal product and raw material used ▶

16 To whom are most of the products or services sold? Please check the appropriate box.   ☐ Business (wholesale)
☐ Public (retail)   ☐ Other (specify) ▶   ☐ N/A

17a Has the applicant ever applied for an identification number for this or any other business? . . . . ☐ Yes ☐ No
Note: *If "Yes," please complete lines 17b and 17c.*

17b If you checked the "Yes" box in line 17a, give applicant's legal name and trade name, if different than name shown on prior application.

Legal name ▶   Trade name ▶

17c Enter approximate date, city, and state where the application was filed and the previous employer identification number if known.
Approximate date when filed (Mo., day, year) City and state where filed

Previous EIN

Under penalties of perjury, I declare that I have examined this application, and to the best of my knowledge and belief, it is true, correct, and complete.

Business telephone number (include area code)

Name and title (Please type or print clearly.) ▶

Signature ▶

Date ▶

Note: *Do not write below this line.   For official use only.*

Please leave blank ▶ | Geo. | Ind. | Class | Size | Reason for applying

For Paperwork Reduction Act Notice, see attached instructions.

Cat. No. 16055N

Form **SS-4** (Rev. 12-93)

General Instructions

(Section references are to the Internal Revenue Code unless otherwise noted.)

Purpose

Use Form SS-4 to apply for an employer identification number (EIN). An EIN is a nine-digit number (for example, 12-3456789) assigned to sole proprietors, corporations, partnerships, estates, trusts, and other entities for filing and reporting purposes. The information you provide on this form will establish your filing and reporting requirements.

Who Must File

You must file this form if you have not obtained an EIN before and

• You pay wages to one or more employees.

• You are required to have an EIN to use on any return, statement, or other document, even if you are not an employer.

• You are a withholding agent required to withhold taxes on income, other than wages, paid to a nonresident alien (individual, corporation, partnership, etc.). A withholding agent may be an agent, broker, fiduciary, manager, tenant, or spouse, and is required to file **Form 1042**, Annual Withholding Tax Return for U.S. Source Income of Foreign Persons.

• You file **Schedule C**, Profit or Loss From Business, or **Schedule F**, Profit or Loss From Farming, of **Form 1040**, U.S. Individual Income Tax Return, and have a Keogh plan or are required to file excise, employment, or alcohol, tobacco, or firearms returns.

The following must use EINs even if they do not have any employees:

• Trusts, except the following:

1. Certain grantor-owned revocable trusts (see the Instructions for Form 1040).

2. Individual Retirement Arrangement (IRA) trusts, unless the trust has to file **Form 990-T**, Exempt Organization Business Income Tax Return (See the Instructions for Form 990-T.)

• Estates

• Partnerships

• REMICS (real estate mortgage investment conduits) (See the instructions for **Form 1066**, U.S. Real Estate Mortgage Investment Conduit Income Tax Return.)

• Corporations

• Nonprofit organizations (churches, clubs, etc.)

• Farmers' cooperatives

• Plan administrators (A plan administrator is the person or group of persons specified as the administrator by the instrument under which the plan is operated.)

Note: *Household employers are not required to file Form SS-4 to get an EIN. An EIN may be assigned to you without filing Form SS-4 if your only employees are household employees (domestic workers) in your private home. To have an EIN assigned to you, write "NONE" in the space for the EIN on* **Form 942**, *Employer's Quarterly Tax Return for Household Employees, when you file it.*

When To Apply for A New EIN

New Business.—If you become the new owner of an existing business, **DO NOT** use the EIN of the former owner. If you already have an EIN, use that number. If you do not have an EIN, apply for one on this form. If you become the "owner" of a corporation by acquiring its stock, use the corporation's EIN.

Changes in Organization or Ownership.—If you already have an EIN, you may need to get a new one if either the organization or ownership of your business changes. If you incorporate a sole proprietorship or form a partnership, you must get a new EIN. However, **DO NOT** apply for a new EIN if you change only the name of your business.

File Only One Form SS-4.—File only one Form SS-4, regardless of the number of businesses operated or trade names under which a business operates. However, each corporation in an affiliated group must file a separate application.

EIN Applied For, But Not Received.—If you do not have an EIN by the time a return is due, write "Applied for" and the date you applied in the space shown for the number. **DO NOT** show your social security number as an EIN on returns.

If you do not have an EIN by the time a tax deposit is due, send your payment to the Internal Revenue service center for your filing area. (See **Where To Apply** below.) Make your check or money order payable to Internal Revenue Service and show your name (as shown on Form SS-4), address, kind of tax, period covered, and date you applied for an EIN.

For more information about EINs, see **Pub. 583**, Taxpayers Starting a Business and **Pub. 1635**, EINs Made Easy.

How To Apply

You can apply for an EIN either by mail or by telephone. You can get an EIN immediately by calling the Tele-TIN phone number for the service center for your state, or you can send the completed Form SS-4 directly to the service center to receive your EIN in the mail.

Application by Tele-TIN.—Under the Tele-TIN program, you can receive your EIN over the telephone and use it immediately to file a return or make a payment. To receive an EIN by phone, complete Form SS-4, then call the Tele-TIN phone number listed for your state under **Where To Apply**. The person making the call must be authorized to sign the form (see **Signature block** on page 3).

An IRS representative will use the information from the Form SS-4 to establish your account and assign you an EIN. Write the number you are given on the upper right-hand corner of the form, sign and date it.

You should mail or FAX the signed SS-4 within 24 hours to the Tele-TIN Unit at the service center address for your state. The IRS representative will give you the FAX number. The FAX numbers are also listed in Pub. 1635.

Taxpayer representatives can receive their client's EIN by phone if they first send a facsimile (FAX) of a completed **Form 2848**, Power of Attorney and Declaration of Representative, or **Form 8821**, Tax Information Authorization, to the Tele-TIN unit. The Form 2848 or Form 8821 will be used solely to release the EIN to the representative authorized on the form.

Application by Mail.—Complete Form SS-4 at least 4 to 5 weeks before you will need an EIN. Sign and date the application and mail it to the service center address for your state. You will receive your EIN in the mail in approximately 4 weeks.

Where To Apply

The Tele-TIN phone numbers listed below will involve a long-distance charge to callers outside of the local calling area, and should be used only to apply for an EIN. THE NUMBERS MAY CHANGE WITHOUT NOTICE. Use 1-800-829-1040 to verify a number or to ask about an application by mail or other Federal tax matters.

If your principal business, office or agency, or legal residence in the case of an individual, is located in: ▼	Call the Tele-TIN phone number shown or file with the Internal Revenue Service center at:
Florida, Georgia, South Carolina	Attn: Entity Control Atlanta, GA 39901 (404) 455-2360
New Jersey, New York City and counties of Nassau, Rockland, Suffolk, and Westchester	Attn: Entity Control Holtsville, NY 00501 (516) 447-4955
New York (all other counties), Connecticut, Maine, Massachusetts, New Hampshire, Rhode Island, Vermont	Attn: Entity Control Andover, MA 05501 (508) 474-9717
Illinois, Iowa, Minnesota, Missouri, Wisconsin	Attn: Entity Control Stop 57A 2306 E. Bannister Rd. Kansas City, MO 64131 (816) 926-5999
Delaware, District of Columbia, Maryland, Pennsylvania, Virginia	Attn: Entity Control Philadelphia, PA 19255 (215) 574-2400

Indiana, Kentucky, Michigan, Ohio, West Virginia	Attn: Entity Control Cincinnati, OH 45999 (606) 292-5467
Kansas, New Mexico, Oklahoma, Texas	Attn: Entity Control Austin, TX 73301 (512) 462-7843
Alaska, Arizona, California (counties of Alpine, Amador, Butte, Calaveras, Colusa, Contra Costa, Del Norte, El Dorado, Glenn, Humboldt, Lake, Lassen, Marin, Mendocino, Modoc, Napa, Nevada, Placer, Plumas, Sacramento, San Joaquin, Shasta, Sierra, Siskiyou, Solano, Sonoma, Sutter, Tehama, Trinity, Yolo, and Yuba), Colorado, Idaho, Montana, Nebraska, Nevada, North Dakota, Oregon, South Dakota, Utah, Washington, Wyoming	Attn: Entity Control Mail Stop 6271-T Ogden, UT 84409 (801) 620-7645
California (all other counties), Hawaii	Attn: Entity Control Fresno, CA 93888 (209) 452-4010
Alabama, Arkansas, Louisiana, Mississippi, North Carolina, Tennessee	Attn: Entity Control Memphis, TN 37501 (901) 365-5970

If you have no legal residence, principal place of business, or principal office or agency in any state, file your form with the Internal Revenue Service Center, Philadelphia, PA 19255 or call (215) 574-2400.

Specific Instructions

The instructions that follow are for those items that are not self-explanatory. Enter N/A (nonapplicable) on the lines that do not apply.

Line 1.—Enter the legal name of the entity applying for the EIN exactly as it appears on the social security card, charter, or other applicable legal document.

Individuals.—Enter the first name, middle initial, and last name.

Trusts.—Enter the name of the trust.

Estate of a decedent.—Enter the name of the estate.

Partnerships.—Enter the legal name of the partnership as it appears in the partnership agreement.

Corporations.—Enter the corporate name as set forth in the corporation charter or other legal document creating it.

Plan administrators.—Enter the name of the plan administrator. A plan administrator who already has an EIN should use that number.

Line 2.—Enter the trade name of the business if different from the legal name. The trade name is the "doing business as" name.

Note: *Use the full legal name on line 1 on all tax returns filed for the entity. However, if you enter a trade name on line 2 and choose to use the trade name instead of the legal name, enter the trade name on all returns you file. To prevent processing delays and errors, **always** use either the legal name only or the trade name only on all tax returns.*

Line 3.—Trusts enter the name of the trustee. Estates enter the name of the executor, administrator, or other fiduciary. If the entity applying has a designated person to receive tax information, enter that person's name as the "care of" person. Print or type the first name, middle initial, and last name.

Line 7.—Enter the first name, middle initial, last name, and social security number (SSN) of a principal officer if the business is a corporation; of a general partner if a partnership; and of a grantor owner, or trustor if a trust.

Line 8a.—Check the box that best describes the type of entity applying for the EIN. If not specifically mentioned, check the "other" box and enter the type of entity. Do not enter N/A.

Sole proprietor.—Check this box if you file Schedule C or F (Form 1040) and have a Keogh plan, or are required to file excise, employment, or alcohol, tobacco, or firearms returns. Enter your SSN (social security number) in the space provided.

Plan administrator.—If the plan administrator is an individual, enter the plan administrator's SSN in the space provided.

Withholding agent.—If you are a withholding agent required to file Form 1042, check the "other" box and enter "withholding agent."

REMICs.—Check this box if the entity has elected to be treated as a real estate mortgage investment conduit (REMIC). See the Instructions for Form 1066 for more information.

Personal service corporations.—Check this box if the entity is a personal service corporation. An entity for a tax year only if:

● The principal activity of the entity during the testing period (prior tax year) for the tax year is the performance of personal services substantially by employee-owners.

● The employee-owners own 10 percent of the fair market value of the outstanding stock of the entity on the last day of the testing period.

Personal services include performance of services in such fields as health, law, accounting, consulting, etc. For more information about personal service corporations, see the instructions for **Form 1120,** U.S. Corporation Income Tax Return, and **Pub. 542,** Tax Information on Corporations.

Other corporations.—This box is for any corporation other than a personal service corporation. If you check this box, enter the type of corporation (such as insurance company) in the space provided.

Other nonprofit organizations.—Check this box if the nonprofit organization is

other than a church or church-controlled organization and specify the type of nonprofit organization (for example, an educational organization.)

If the organization also seeks tax-exempt status, you must file either **Package 1023** or **Package 1024,** Application for Recognition of Exemption. Get **Pub. 557,** Tax-Exempt Status for Your Organization, for more information.

Group exemption number (GEN).—If the organization is covered by a group exemption letter, enter the four-digit GEN. (Do not confuse the GEN with the nine-digit EIN.) If you do not know the GEN, contact the parent organization. Get Pub. 557 for more information about group exemption numbers.

Line 9.—Check only **one** box. Do not enter N/A.

Started new business.—Check this box if you are starting a new business that requires an EIN. If you check this box, enter the type of business being started. **DO NOT** apply if you already have an EIN and are only adding another place of business.

Changed type of organization.—Check this box if the business is changing its type of organization, for example, if the business was a sole proprietorship and has been incorporated or has become a partnership. If you check this box, specify in the space provided the type of change made, for example, "from sole proprietorship to partnership."

Purchased going business.—Check this box if you purchased an existing business. DO NOT use the former owner's EIN. Use your own EIN if you already have one.

Hired employees.—Check this box if the existing business is requesting an EIN because it has hired or is hiring employees and is therefore required to file employment tax returns. **DO NOT** apply if you already have an EIN and are only hiring employees. If you are hiring household employees, see **Note** under **Who Must File** on page 2.

Created a trust.—Check this box if you created a trust, and enter the type of trust created.

Note: *DO NOT file this form if you are the individual-grantor/owner of a revocable trust. You must use your SSN for the trust. See the instructions for Form 1040.*

Created a pension plan.—Check this box if you have created a pension plan and need this number for reporting purposes. Also, enter the type of plan created.

Banking purpose.—Check this box if you are requesting an EIN for banking purposes only and enter the banking purpose (for example, a bowling league for depositing dues, an investment club for dividend and interest reporting, etc.).

Other (specify).—Check this box if you are requesting an EIN for any reason other than those for which there are checkboxes, and enter the reason.

Line 10.—If you are starting a new business, enter the starting date of the business. If the business you acquired is already operating, enter the date you acquired the business. Trusts should enter the date the trust was legally created. Estates should enter the date of death of the decedent whose name appears on line 1 or the date when the estate was legally funded.

Line 11.—Enter the last month of your accounting year or tax year. An accounting or tax year is usually 12 consecutive months, either a calendar year or a fiscal year (including a period of 52 or 53 weeks). A calendar year is 12 consecutive months ending on December 31. A fiscal year is either 12 consecutive months ending on the last day of any month other than December or a 52-53 week year. For more information on accounting periods, see **Pub. 538,** Accounting Periods and Methods.

Individuals.—Your tax year generally will be a calendar year.

Partnerships.—Partnerships generally must adopt the tax year of either (1) the majority partners; (2) the principal partners; (3) the tax year that results in the least aggregate (total) deferral of income; or (4) some other tax year. (See the Instructions for **Form 1065,** U.S. Partnership Return of Income, for more information.)

REMICs.—Remics must have a calendar year as their tax year.

Personal service corporations.—A personal service corporation generally must adopt a calendar year unless:

• It can establish a business purpose for having a different tax year, or

• It elects under section 444 to have a tax year other than a calendar year.

Trusts.—Generally, a trust must adopt a calendar year except for the following:

• Tax-exempt trusts,

• Charitable trusts, and

• Grantor-owned trusts.

Line 12.—If the business has or will have employees, enter the date on which the business began or will begin to pay wages. If the business does not plan to have employees, enter N/A.

Withholding agent.—Enter the date you began or will begin to pay income to a nonresident alien. This also applies to individuals who are required to file Form 1042 to report alimony paid to a nonresident alien.

Line 14.—Generally, enter the exact type of business being operated (for example, advertising agency, farm, food or beverage establishment, labor union, real estate agency, steam laundry, rental of coin-operated vending machine, investment club, etc.). Also state if the business will involve the sale or distribution of alcoholic beverages.

Governmental.—Enter the type of organization (state, county, school district, or municipality, etc.).

Nonprofit organization (other than governmental).—Enter whether organized for religious, educational, or humane purposes, and the principal activity (for example, religious organization—hospital, charitable).

Mining and quarrying.—Specify the process and the principal product (for example, mining bituminous coal, contract drilling for oil, quarrying dimension stone, etc.).

Contract construction.—Specify whether general contracting or special trade contracting. Also, show the type of work normally performed (for example, general contractor for residential buildings, electrical subcontractor, etc.).

Food or beverage establishments.—Specify the type of establishment and state whether you employ workers who receive tips (for example, lounge—yes).

Trade.—Specify the type of sales and the principal line of goods sold (for example, wholesale dairy products, manufacturer's representative for mining machinery, retail hardware, etc.).

Manufacturing.—Specify the type of establishment operated (for example, sawmill, vegetable cannery, etc.).

Signature block.—The application must be signed by: (1) the individual, if the applicant is an individual, (2) the president, vice president, or other principal officer, if the applicant is a corporation, (3) a responsible and duly authorized member or officer having knowledge of its affairs, if the applicant is a partnership or other unincorporated organization, or (4) the fiduciary, if the applicant is a trust or estate.

Some Useful Publications

You may get the following publications for additional information on the subjects covered on this form. To get these and other free forms and publications, call 1-800-TAX-FORM (1-800-829-3676).

Pub. 1635, EINs Made Easy

Pub. 538, Accounting Periods and Methods

Pub. 541, Tax Information on Partnerships

Pub. 542, Tax Information on Corporations

Pub. 557, Tax-Exempt Status for Your Organization

Pub. 583, Taxpayers Starting A Business

Pub. 937, Employment Taxes and Information Returns

Package 1023, Application for Recognition of Exemption

Package 1024, Application for Recognition of Exemption Under Section 501(a) or for Determination Under Section 120

Paperwork Reduction Act Notice

We ask for the information on this form to carry out the Internal Revenue laws of the United States. You are required to give us the information. We need it to ensure that you are complying with these laws and to allow us to figure and collect the right amount of tax.

The time needed to complete and file this form will vary depending on individual circumstances. The estimated average time is:

Recordkeeping . . . . . . 7 min.

Learning about the law or the form . . . . . 18 min.

Preparing the form . . . . 44 min.

Copying, assembling, and sending the form to the IRS . 20 min.

If you have comments concerning the accuracy of these time estimates or suggestions for making this form more simple, we would be happy to hear from you. You can write to both the **Internal Revenue Service,** Attention: Reports Clearance Officer, PC:FP, Washington, DC 20224; and the **Office of Management and Budget,** Paperwork Reduction Project (1545-0003), Washington, DC 20503. **DO NOT** send this form to either of these offices. Instead, see **Where To Apply** on page 2.

 Printed on recycled paper

*U.S. Government Printing Office: 1993 — 363-331/99125

Form W-4 (1995)

Want More Money In Your Paycheck?
If you expect to be able to take the earned income credit for 1995 and a child lives with you, you may be able to have part of the credit added to your take-home pay. For details, get Form W-5 from your employer.

Purpose. Complete Form W-4 so that your employer can withhold the correct amount of Federal income tax from your pay.

Exemption From Withholding. Read line 7 of the certificate below to see if you can claim exempt status. If exempt, complete line 7; but do not complete lines 5 and 6. No Federal income tax will be withheld from your pay. Your exemption is good for 1 year only. It expires February 15, 1996.

Note: You cannot claim exemption from withholding if (1) your income exceeds $650 and includes unearned income (e.g., interest

and dividends) and (2) another person can claim you as a dependent on their tax return.

Basic Instructions. Employees who are not exempt should complete the Personal Allowances Worksheet. Additional worksheets are provided on page 2 for employees to adjust their withholding allowances based on itemized deductions, adjustments to income, or two-earner/two-job situations. Complete all worksheets that apply to your situation. The worksheets will help you figure the number of withholding allowances you are entitled to claim. However, you may claim fewer allowances than this.

Head of Household. Generally, you may claim head of household filing status on your tax return only if you are unmarried and pay more than 50% of the costs of keeping up a home for yourself and your dependent(s) or other qualifying individuals.

Nonwage Income. If you have a large amount of nonwage income, such as interest or dividends, you should consider making

estimated tax payments using Form 1040-ES. Otherwise, you may find that you owe additional tax at the end of the year.

Two Earners/Two Jobs. If you have a working spouse or more than one job, figure the total number of allowances you are entitled to claim on all jobs using worksheets from only one Form W-4. This total should be divided among all jobs. Your withholding will usually be most accurate when all allowances are claimed on the W-4 filed for the highest paying job and zero allowances are claimed for the others.

Check Your Withholding. After your W-4 takes effect, you can use **Pub. 919,** Is My Withholding Correct for 1995?, to see how the dollar amount you are having withheld compares to your estimated total annual tax. We recommend you get Pub. 919 especially if you used the Two Earner/Two Job Worksheet and your earnings exceed $150,000 (Single) or $200,000 (Married). Call 1-800-829-3676 to order Pub. 919. Check your telephone directory for the IRS assistance number for further help.

Personal Allowances Worksheet

A Enter "1" for **yourself** if no one else can claim you as a dependent . . . . **A** _____

B Enter "1" if:
- You are single and have only one job; or
- You are married, have only one job, and your spouse does not work; or
- Your wages from a second job or your spouse's wages (or the total of both) are $1,000 or less.
. . **B** _____

C Enter "1" for your **spouse.** But, you may choose to enter -0- if you are married and have either a working spouse or more than one job (this may help you avoid having too little tax withheld) . . . . **C** _____

D Enter number of **dependents** (other than your spouse or yourself) you will claim on your tax return . . . . . . **D** _____

E Enter "1" if you will file as **head of household** on your tax return (see conditions under **Head of Household** above) . . **E** _____

F Enter "1" if you have at least $1,500 of **child or dependent care expenses** for which you plan to claim a credit . . **F** _____

G Add lines A through F and enter total here. **Note:** This amount may be different from the number of exemptions you claim on your return ▶ **G** _____

For accuracy, do all worksheets that apply.	• If you plan to **itemize or claim adjustments to income** and want to reduce your withholding, see the Deductions and Adjustments Worksheet on page 2.
	• If you are **single** and have **more than one job** and your combined earnings from all jobs exceed $30,000 **OR** if you are **married** and have a **working spouse** or **more than one job,** and the combined earnings from all jobs exceed $50,000, see the Two-Earner/Two-Job Worksheet on page 2 if you want to avoid having too little tax withheld.
	• If **neither** of the above situations applies, **stop here** and enter the number from line G on line 5 of Form W-4 below.

- - - - - - - - **Cut here and give the certificate to your employer. Keep the top portion for your records.** - - - - - - - -

---

Form **W-4**
Department of the Treasury
Internal Revenue Service

Employee's Withholding Allowance Certificate

▶ **For Privacy Act and Paperwork Reduction Act Notice, see reverse.**

OMB No. 1545-0010

1995

1 Type or print your first name and middle initial	Last name	2 Your social security number

Home address (number and street or rural route)	3 ☐ Single ☐ Married ☐ Married, but withhold at higher Single rate. **Note:** If married, but legally separated, or spouse is a nonresident alien, check the Single box.

City or town, state, and ZIP code	4 If your last name differs from that on your social security card, check here and call 1-800-772-1213 for a new card . . . . . ▶ ☐

5 Total number of allowances you are claiming (from line G above or from the worksheets on page 2 if they apply) . **5** _____

6 Additional amount, if any, you want withheld from each paycheck . . . . **6** $ _____

7 I claim exemption from withholding for 1995 and I certify that I meet **BOTH** of the following conditions for exemption:
- Last year I had a right to a refund of **ALL** Federal income tax withheld because I had **NO** tax liability; **AND**
- This year I expect a refund of **ALL** Federal income tax withheld because I expect to have **NO** tax liability.

If you meet both conditions, enter "EXEMPT" here . . . . ▶ **7** _____

Under penalties of perjury, I certify that I am entitled to the number of withholding allowances claimed on this certificate or entitled to claim exempt status.

Employee's signature ▶ _____ **Date** ▶ _____, 19__

8 Employer's name and address (Employer: Complete 8 and 10 only if sending to the IRS)	9 Office code (optional)	10 Employer identification number

Cat. No. 10220Q

Deductions and Adjustments Worksheet

Note: *Use this worksheet only if you plan to itemize deductions or claim adjustments to income on your 1995 tax return.*

1　Enter an estimate of your 1995 itemized deductions. These include qualifying home mortgage interest, charitable contributions, state and local taxes (but not sales taxes), medical expenses in excess of 7.5% of your income, and miscellaneous deductions. (For 1995, you may have to reduce your itemized deductions if your income is over $114,700 ($57,350 if married filing separately). Get Pub. 919 for details.)　**1** $ _____

2　Enter: $\left\{\begin{array}{l}\text{\$6,550 if married filing jointly or qualifying widow(er)}\\ \text{\$5,750 if head of household}\\ \text{\$3,900 if single}\\ \text{\$3,275 if married filing separately}\end{array}\right\}$ . . . .　**2** $ _____

3　**Subtract** line 2 from line 1. If line 2 is greater than line 1, enter -0- . . . . . .　**3** $ _____

4　Enter an estimate of your 1995 adjustments to income. These include alimony paid and deductible IRA contributions　**4** $ _____

5　**Add** lines 3 and 4 and enter the total . . . .　**5** $ _____

6　Enter an estimate of your 1995 nonwage income (such as dividends or interest) . . . . .　**6** $ _____

7　**Subtract** line 6 from line 5. Enter the result, but not less than -0- . . . .　**7** $ _____

8　**Divide** the amount on line 7 by $2,500 and enter the result here. Drop any fraction . . . .　**8** _____

9　Enter the number from Personal Allowances Worksheet, line G, on page 1 . . . .　**9** _____

10　**Add** lines 8 and 9 and enter the total here. If you plan to use the Two-Earner/Two-Job Worksheet, also enter this total on line 1 below. Otherwise, **stop here** and enter this total on Form W-4, line 5, on page 1 . . . . .　**10** _____

Two-Earner/Two-Job Worksheet

Note: *Use this worksheet only if the instructions for line G on page 1 direct you here.*

1　Enter the number from line G on page 1 (or from line 10 above if you used the Deductions and Adjustments Worksheet)　**1** _____

2　Find the number in **Table 1** below that applies to the **LOWEST** paying job and enter it here . . . .　**2** _____

3　If line 1 is **GREATER THAN OR EQUAL TO** line 2, subtract line 2 from line 1. Enter the result here (if zero, enter -0-) and on Form W-4, line 5, on page 1. **DO NOT** use the rest of this worksheet . . . .　**3** _____

Note: *If line 1 is **LESS THAN** line 2, enter -0- on Form W-4, line 5, on page 1. Complete lines 4–9 to calculate the additional withholding amount necessary to avoid a year end tax bill.*

4　Enter the number from line 2 of this worksheet . . . .　**4** _____

5　Enter the number from line 1 of this worksheet . . . .　**5** _____

6　**Subtract** line 5 from line 4 . . . .　**6** _____

7　Find the amount in **Table 2** below that applies to the **HIGHEST** paying job and enter it here . . . .　**7** $ _____

8　**Multiply** line 7 by line 6 and enter the result here. This is the additional annual withholding amount needed　**8** $ _____

9　Divide line 8 by the number of pay periods remaining in 1995. (For example, divide by 26 if you are paid every other week and you complete this form in December 1994.) Enter the result here and on Form W-4, line 6, page 1. This is the additional amount to be withheld from each paycheck . . . .　**9** $ _____

Table 1: Two-Earner/Two-Job Worksheet

Married Filing Jointly				All Others	
If wages from **LOWEST** paying job are—	Enter on line 2 above	If wages from **LOWEST** paying job are—	Enter on line 2 above	If wages from **LOWEST** paying job are—	Enter on line 2 above
0 - $3,000	0	39,001 - 50,000	9	0 - $4,000	0
3,001 - 6,000	1	50,001 - 55,000	10	4,001 - 10,000	1
6,001 - 11,000	2	55,001 - 60,000	11	10,001 - 14,000	2
11,001 - 16,000	3	60,001 - 70,000	12	14,001 - 19,000	3
16,001 - 21,000	4	70,001 - 80,000	13	19,001 - 23,000	4
21,001 - 27,000	5	80,001 - 90,000	14	23,001 - 45,000	5
27,001 - 31,000	6	90,001 and over	15	45,001 - 60,000	6
31,001 - 34,000	7			60,001 - 70,000	7
34,001 - 39,000	8			70,001 and over	8

Table 2: Two-Earner/Two-Job Worksheet

Married Filing Jointly		All Others	
If wages from **HIGHEST** paying job are—	Enter on line 7 above	If wages from **HIGHEST** paying job are—	Enter on line 7 above
0 - $50,000	$380	0 - $30,000	$380
50,001 - 100,000	700	30,001 - 60,000	700
100,001 - 130,000	780	60,001 - 110,000	780
130,001 - 230,000	900	110,001 - 230,000	900
230,001 and over	990	230,001 and over	990

Privacy Act and Paperwork Reduction Act Notice.—We ask for the information on this form to carry out the Internal Revenue laws of the United States. The Internal Revenue Code requires this information under sections 3402(f)(2)(A) and 6109 and their regulations. Failure to provide a completed form will result in your being treated as a single person who claims no withholding allowances. Routine uses of this information include giving it to the Department of Justice for civil and criminal litigation and to cities, states, and the District of Columbia for use in administering their tax laws.

The time needed to complete this form will vary depending on individual circumstances. The estimated average time is: **Recordkeeping** 46 min., **Learning about the law or the form** 10 min., **Preparing the form** 69 min. If you have comments concerning the accuracy of these time estimates or suggestions for making this form simpler, we would be happy to hear from you. You can write to the **Internal Revenue Service**, Attention: Tax Forms Committee, PC:FP, Washington, DC 20224. **DO NOT** send the tax form to this address. Instead, give it to your employer.

 Printed on recycled paper　　　　　　　　　　　　*U.S. Government Printing Office: 1994 — 375-119*

U.S. Department of Justice
Immigration and Naturalization Service

OMB No. 1115-0136
Employment Eligibility Verification

Please read instructions carefully before completing this form. The instructions must be available during completion of this form. **ANTI-DISCRIMINATION NOTICE.** It is illegal to discriminate against work eligible individuals. Employers CANNOT specify which document(s) they will accept from an employee. The refusal to hire an individual because of a future expiration date may also constitute illegal discrimination.

Section 1. Employee Information and Verification. To be completed and signed by employee at the time employment begins

Print Name: Last	First	Middle Initial	Maiden Name

Address (Street Name and Number)	Apt. #	Date of Birth (month/day/year)

City	State	Zip Code	Social Security #

I am aware that federal law provides for imprisonment and/or fines for false statements or use of false documents in connection with the completion of this form.

I attest, under penalty of perjury, that I am (check one of the following):
- ☐ A citizen or national of the United States
- ☐ A Lawful Permanent Resident (Alien # A _____)
- ☐ An alien authorized to work until ___/___/___ (Alien # or Admission # _____)

Employee's Signature	Date (month/day/year)

Preparer and/or Translator Certification. (To be completed and signed if Section 1 is prepared by a person other than the employee.) I attest, under penalty of perjury, that I have assisted in the completion of this form and that to the best of my knowledge the information is true and correct.

Preparer's/Translator's Signature	Print Name

Address (Street Name and Number, City, State, Zip Code)	Date (month/day/year)

Section 2. Employer Review and Verification. To be completed and signed by employer. Examine one document from List A OR examine one document from List B and one from List C as listed on the reverse of this form and record the title, number and expiration date, if any, of the document(s)

List A	OR	List B	AND	List C
Document title:				
Issuing authority:				
Document #:				
Expiration Date (if any): ___/___/___		___/___/___		___/___/___
Document #:				
Expiration Date (if any): ___/___/___				

CERTIFICATION - I attest, under penalty of perjury, that I have examined the document(s) presented by the above-named employee, that the above-listed document(s) appear to be genuine and to relate to the employee named, that the employee began employment on (month/day/year) ___/___/___ **and that to the best of my knowledge the employee is eligible to work in the United States.** (State employment agencies may omit the date the employee began employment).

Signature of Employer or Authorized Representative	Print Name	Title

Business or Organization Name	Address (Street Name and Number, City, State, Zip Code)	Date (month/day/year)

Section 3. Updating and Reverification. To be completed and signed by employer

A. New Name (if applicable)	B. Date of rehire (month/day/year) (if applicable)

C. If employee's previous grant of work authorization has expired, provide the information below for the document that establishes current employment eligibility.

Document Title:_____ Document #:_____ Expiration Date (if any): ___/___/___

I attest, under penalty of perjury, that to the best of my knowledge, this employee is eligible to work in the United States, and if the employee presented document(s), the document(s) I have examined appear to be genuine and to relate to the individual.

Signature of Employer or Authorized Representative	Date (month/day/year)

Form I-9 (Rev. 11-21-91) N

LISTS OF ACCEPTABLE DOCUMENTS

LIST A		LIST B		LIST C
Documents that Establish Both Identity and Employment Eligibility	**OR**	**Documents that Establish Identity**	**AND**	**Documents that Establish Employment Eligibility**

LIST A — Documents that Establish Both Identity and Employment Eligibility

1. U.S. Passport (unexpired or expired)

2. Certificate of U.S. Citizenship *(INS Form N-560 or N-561)*

3. Certificate of Naturalization *(INS Form N-550 or N-570)*

4. Unexpired foreign passport, with *I-551 stamp* or attached INS Form *I-94* indicating unexpired employment authorization

5. Alien Registration Receipt Card with photograph *(INS Form I-151 or I-551)*

6. Unexpired Temporary Resident Card *(INS Form I-688)*

7. Unexpired Employment Authorization Card *(INS Form I-688A)*

8. Unexpired Reentry Permit *(INS Form I-327)*

9. Unexpired Refugee Travel Document *(INS Form I-571)*

10. Unexpired Employment Authorization Document issued by the INS which contains a photograph *(INS Form I-688B)*

LIST B — Documents that Establish Identity

1. Driver's license or ID card issued by a state or outlying possession of the United States provided it contains a photograph or information such as name, date of birth, sex, height, eye color, and address

2. ID card issued by federal, state, or local government agencies or entities provided it contains a photograph or information such as name, date of birth, sex, height, eye color, and address

3. School ID card with a photograph

4. Voter's registration card

5. U.S. Military card or draft record

6. Military dependent's ID card

7. U.S. Coast Guard Merchant Mariner Card

8. Native American tribal document

9. Driver's license issued by a Canadian government authority

For persons under age 18 who are unable to present a document listed above:

10. School record or report card

11. Clinic, doctor, or hospital record

12. Day-care or nursery school record

LIST C — Documents that Establish Employment Eligibility

1. U.S. social security card issued by the Social Security Administration *(other than a card stating it is not valid for employment)*

2. Certification of Birth Abroad issued by the Department of State *(Form FS-545 or Form DS-1350)*

3. Original or certified copy of a birth certificate issued by a state, county, municipal authority or outlying possession of the United States bearing an official seal

4. Native American tribal document

5. U.S. Citizen ID Card *(INS Form I-197)*

6. ID Card for use of Resident Citizen in the United States *(INS Form I-179)*

7. Unexpired employment authorization document issued by the INS *(other than those listed under List A)*

Illustrations of many of these documents appear in Part 8 of the Handbook for Employers (M-274)

Form I-9 (Rev. 11-21-91) N

FPI-RBK

☆ U.S. GPO:1993-301-643/92153

a Control number	22222	Void ☐	For Official Use Only ► OMB No. 1545-0008	

b Employer's identification number		**1** Wages, tips, other compensation	**2** Federal income tax withheld
c Employer's name, address, and ZIP code		**3** Social security wages	**4** Social security tax withheld
		5 Medicare wages and tips	**6** Medicare tax withheld
		7 Social security tips	**8** Allocated tips
d Employee's social security number		**9** Advance EIC payment	**10** Dependent care benefits
e Employee's name (first, middle initial, last)		**11** Nonqualified plans	**12** Benefits included in box 1
		13 See Instrs. for box 13	**14** Other

15 Statutory employee ☐ Deceased ☐ Pension plan ☐ Legal rep. ☐ 942 emp. ☐ Subtotal ☐ Deferred compensation ☐

f Employee's address and ZIP code						
16 State Employer's state I.D. No.	**17** State wages, tips, etc.	**18** State income tax	**19** Locality name	**20** Local wages, tips, etc.	**21** Local income tax

Cat. No. 10134D   Department of the Treasury—Internal Revenue Service

Form **W-2** Wage and Tax Statement **1994**

For Paperwork Reduction Act Notice, see separate instructions.

Copy A For Social Security Administration

Do NOT Cut or Separate Forms on This Page

---

a Control number	22222	Void ☐	For Official Use Only ► OMB No. 1545-0008	

b Employer's identification number		**1** Wages, tips, other compensation	**2** Federal income tax withheld
c Employer's name, address, and ZIP code		**3** Social security wages	**4** Social security tax withheld
		5 Medicare wages and tips	**6** Medicare tax withheld
		7 Social security tips	**8** Allocated tips
d Employee's social security number		**9** Advance EIC payment	**10** Dependent care benefits
e Employee's name (first, middle initial, last)		**11** Nonqualified plans	**12** Benefits included in box 1
		13 See Instrs. for box 13	**14** Other

15 Statutory employee ☐ Deceased ☐ Pension plan ☐ Legal rep. ☐ 942 emp. ☐ Subtotal ☐ Deferred compensation ☐

f Employee's address and ZIP code						
16 State Employer's state I.D. No.	**17** State wages, tips, etc.	**18** State income tax	**19** Locality name	**20** Local wages, tips, etc.	**21** Local income tax

Cat. No. 10134D   Department of the Treasury—Internal Revenue Service

Form **W-2** Wage and Tax Statement **1994**

For Paperwork Reduction Act Notice, see separate instructions.

Copy A For Social Security Administration

Form **940-EZ**

Department of the Treasury
Internal Revenue Service (O)

Employer's Annual Federal
Unemployment (FUTA) Tax Return

1994

OMB No. 1545-1110

T	
FF	
FD	
FP	
I	
T	

Name (as distinguished from trade name)   Calendar year

Trade name, if any

Address and ZIP code   Employer identification number

*Follow the chart under **Who May Use Form 940-EZ** on page 2. If you cannot use Form 940-EZ, you must use Form 940 instead.*

A Enter the amount of contributions paid to your state unemployment fund. (See instructions for line A on page 4.) ▶ $ ....

B (1) Enter the name of the state where you have to pay contributions . . . . ▶ ....

   (2) Enter your state reporting number as shown on state unemployment tax return. ▶

If you will not have to file returns in the future, check here (see Who Must File, on page 2) **complete, and sign the return** . . . . . ▶ ☐

If this is an Amended Return check here . . . . ▶ ☐

Part I   Taxable Wages and FUTA Tax

1 Total payments (including payments shown on lines 2 and 3) during the calendar year for services of employees | **1** |

Amount paid

2 Exempt payments. (Explain all exempt payments, attaching additional sheets if necessary.) ▶ ....

.... | **2** |

3 Payments for services of more than $7,000. Enter only amounts over the first $7,000 paid to each employee. Do not include any exempt payments from line 2. Do not use your state wage limitation. The $7,000 amount is the Federal wage base. Your state wage base may be different . . . . | **3** |

4 Total exempt payments (add lines 2 and 3) . . . . | **4** |

5 **Total taxable wages** (subtract line 4 from line 1) . . . . ▶ | **5** |

6 **FUTA tax.** Multiply the wages on line 5 by .008 and enter here. (If the result is over $100, also complete Part II.) . | **6** |

7 Total FUTA tax deposited for the year, including any overpayment applied from a prior year (from your records) . | **7** |

8 **Amount you owe** (subtract line 7 from line 6). This should be $100 or less. Pay to "Internal Revenue Service." ▶ | **8** |

9 **Overpayment** (subtract line 6 from line 7). Check if it is to be: ☐ **Applied to next return, or** ☐ **Refunded** ▶ | **9** |

Part II   Record of Quarterly Federal Unemployment Tax Liability (Do not include state liability.) Complete only if line 6 is over $100.

Quarter	First (Jan. 1 – Mar. 31)	Second (Apr. 1 – June 30)	Third (July 1 – Sept. 30)	Fourth (Oct. 1 – Dec. 31)	Total for year
Liability for quarter					

Under penalties of perjury, I declare that I have examined this return, including accompanying schedules and statements, and, to the best of my knowledge and belief, it is true, correct, and complete, and that no part of any payment made to a state unemployment fund claimed as a credit was, or is to be, deducted from the payments to employees.

Signature ▶   Title (Owner, etc.) ▶   Date ▶

Cat. No. 10983G   Form **940-EZ** (1994)

DO NOT DETACH

- -

Form **940-V-EZ**

Department of the Treasury
Internal Revenue Service

Form 940-EZ Payment Voucher

1994

Complete boxes 1, 2, 6, and 7. **Do not send cash and do not staple your payment to this voucher.** Make your check or money order, with your employer identification number clearly written on it, payable to the **Internal Revenue Service.**

1 Your employer identification number	2 Enter the first four letters of your business name	3 MFT	4 Tax year	5 Transaction code
		1 0	9 4 1 2	6 1 0
	6 Your name and address		7 Amount of payment	
			$	.
Do not staple your payment to this voucher.			Do not send cash.	

Paperwork Reduction Act Notice.—We ask for the information on this form to carry out the Internal Revenue laws of the United States. You are required to give us the information. We need it to ensure that you are complying with these laws and to allow us to figure and collect the correct tax.

The time needed to complete and file this form will vary depending on individual circumstances. The estimated average time is:

Recordkeeping . . . . 6 hr., 23 min.
**Learning about the
law or the form** . . . . 7 min.

**Preparing and sending
the form to the IRS** . . . . 34 min.

If you have comments concerning the accuracy of these time estimates or suggestions for making this form simpler, we would be happy to hear from you. You can write to both the **Internal Revenue Service**, Attention: Tax Forms Committee, PC:FP, Washington, DC 20224; and the **Office of Management and Budget**, Paperwork Reduction Project (1545-1110), Washington, DC 20503. **DO NOT** send the form to either of these offices. Instead, see **Where To File** on page 4.

Who May Use Form 940-EZ

The following chart will lead you to the right form to use.

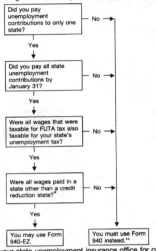

* Contact your state unemployment insurance office for credit reduction state information.

** If you need to file Form 940, you can get the form by calling 1-800-829-3676 (1-800-TAX-FORM).

Note: Do not file Form 940-EZ if you have already filed Form 940 for 1994.

General Instructions

Purpose of Form.—Use this form to report your annual Federal Unemployment Tax Act (FUTA) tax. FUTA tax, together with state unemployment systems, provides for payments of unemployment compensation to workers who have lost their jobs. Most employers pay both Federal and state unemployment taxes. **Only the employer pays this tax.** The tax applies to the first $7,000 you pay each employee in a year. The $7,000 amount is the Federal wage base. Your state wage base may be different.

When To File.—Form 940-EZ for 1994 is due by January 31, 1995. However, if you deposited all FUTA tax when due, you may file on or before February 10.

Who Must File

General Rule (household and agricultural employers see below).—File if either of the following applies:

1. You paid wages of $1,500 or more in any calendar quarter in 1993 or 1994; or

2. You had at least one employee for some part of a day in any 20 different weeks in 1993 or 1994.

Count all regular, temporary, and part-time employees. A partnership should not count its partners. If a business changes hands during the year, each employer meeting test 1 or 2 must file. Do not report wages paid by the other.

Household Employers.—File a FUTA tax return **ONLY** if you paid cash wages of $1,000 or more in any calendar quarter in 1993 or 1994 for household work in a private home, local college club, or a local chapter of a college fraternity or sorority.

Note: See **Pub. 926**, Employment Taxes for Household Employers, for more information including filled-in examples of Form 940-EZ.

Agricultural Employers.—File a FUTA tax return if either of the following applies:

1. You paid cash wages of $20,000 or more to farmworkers during any calendar quarter in 1993 or 1994; or

2. You employed 10 or more farmworkers during some part of a day (whether or not at the same time) for at least 1 day during any 20 different weeks in 1993 or 1994.

Count aliens admitted on a temporary basis to the United States to perform farmwork, also known as workers with "H-2(a)" visas, to see if you meet either test. Wages paid to these aliens are not subject to FUTA tax before 1995.

Nonprofit Organizations.—Religious, educational, charitable, etc., organizations described in section 501(c)(3) of the Internal Revenue Code and exempt from tax under section 501(a) are not subject to FUTA tax and are not required to file.

(Instructions continued on next page.)

Form **940-EZ**		
Department of the Treasury Internal Revenue Service	**Employer's Annual Federal Unemployment (FUTA) Tax Return**	OMB No. 1545-1110 **1994**

Name (as distinguished from trade name)

Trade name, if any

Address and ZIP code

Employer identification number

*Follow the chart under **Who May Use Form 940-EZ** on page 2. If you cannot use Form 940-EZ, you must use Form 940 instead.*

A Enter the amount of contributions paid to your state unemployment fund. (See instructions for line A on page 4.) ▶ $ ....

B (1) Enter the name of the state where you have to pay contributions . . . . ▶ ....

    (2) Enter your state reporting number as shown on state unemployment tax return. ▶ ....

If you will not have to file returns in the future, check here (see **Who Must File**, on page 2) **complete, and sign the return** . . . . . . ▶ ☐

If this is an Amended Return check here . . . . ▶ ☐

Part I   **Taxable Wages and FUTA Tax**

1	Total payments (including payments shown on lines 2 and 3) during the calendar year for services of employees	**1**
2	Exempt payments. (Explain all exempt payments, attaching additional sheets if necessary.) ▶	**2** Amount paid
3	Payments for services of more than $7,000. Enter only amounts over the first $7,000 paid to each employee. Do not include any exempt payments from line 2. Do not use your state wage limitation. The $7,000 amount is the Federal wage base. Your state wage base may be different	**3**
4	Total exempt payments (add lines 2 and 3)	**4**
5	**Total taxable wages** (subtract line 4 from line 1) . . . . ▶	**5**
6	**FUTA tax.** Multiply the wages on line 5 by .008 and enter here. (If the result is over $100, also complete Part II.) .	**6**
7	Total FUTA tax deposited for the year, including any overpayment applied from a prior year (from your records)	**7**
8	**Amount you owe** (subtract line 7 from line 6). This should be $100 or less. Pay to "Internal Revenue Service." ▶	**8**
9	**Overpayment** (subtract line 6 from line 7). Check if it is to be: ☐ **Applied to next return, or** ☐ **Refunded** ▶	**9**

Part II   **Record of Quarterly Federal Unemployment Tax Liability** (Do not include state liability.) Complete only if line 6 is over $100.

Quarter	First (Jan. 1 – Mar. 31)	Second (Apr. 1 – June 30)	Third (July 1 – Sept. 30)	Fourth (Oct. 1 – Dec. 31)	Total for year
Liability for quarter					

Under penalties of perjury, I declare that I have examined this return, including accompanying schedules and statements, and, to the best of my knowledge and belief, it is true, correct, and complete, and that no part of any payment made to a state unemployment fund claimed as a credit was, or is to be, deducted from the payments to employees.

Signature ▶   Title (Owner, etc.) ▶   Date ▶

Form **940-EZ** (1994)

Completing Form 940-EZ.—If your FUTA tax for 1994 (line 6) is $100 or less, complete only Part I of the form. If your FUTA tax is over $100, complete Parts I and II. See the instructions for Part II for information on FUTA tax deposits.

If You Are Not Liable for FUTA Tax.—If you receive Form 940-EZ and are not liable for FUTA tax for 1994, write "Not Liable" across the front of the form, sign the return, and return it to the IRS.
Note: *If you will not have to file returns in the future, check the box on the line below B(2), complete and sign the return.*

Employer's Name, Address, and Identification Number.—If you are not using a preaddressed Form 940-EZ, type or print your name, trade name, address, and employer identification number (EIN) on Form 940-EZ.

See **Pub. 937,** Employment Taxes, for details on how to make tax deposits, file a return, etc., if these are due before you get your EIN.

Identifying Your Payments.—When you pay any amount you owe to the IRS (line 8) or make Federal tax deposits, write the following on your check or money order: your EIN, "Form 940-EZ," and the tax period to which the payment applies. This helps make sure we credit your account properly.

Penalties and Interest.—Avoid penalties and interest by making tax deposits when due, filing a correct return, and paying all taxes

when due. There are penalties for late deposits and late filing unless you can show reasonable cause. If you file late, attach an explanation to the return.

There are also penalties for willful failure to pay tax, keep records, make returns, and for filing false or fraudulent returns.
Credit for Contributions Paid Into State Funds.—You get a credit for amounts you pay to a state (including Puerto Rico) unemployment fund by January 31. This credit is reflected in the FUTA tax rate (.008) shown on line 6. The rate is effective through 1998.

"Contributions" are payments that a state requires you, as an employer, to make to its unemployment fund for the payment of unemployment benefits. However, contributions do not include:

● Any payments deducted or deductible from your employees' pay.

● Penalties, interest, or special administrative taxes not included in the contribution rate the state assigned to you.

● Voluntary contributions you paid to get a lower assigned rate.
Note: *Be sure to enter your state reporting number on line B(2) at the top of the form. We need this to verify your state contributions.*
Credit for Successor Employers.—If you are claiming credit as a successor employer, you must use Form 940.

(Instructions continued on next page.)

Where To File.—In the list below, find the state where your legal residence, principal place of business, office, or agency is located. Send your return to the **Internal Revenue Service** at the address listed for your location. No street address is needed.

Note: *Where you file depends on whether or not you are including a payment.*

Florida, Georgia, South Carolina

Return without payment:	Return with payment:
Atlanta, GA 39901-0047	P.O. Box 105659
	Atlanta, GA 30348-5659

New Jersey, New York (New York City and counties of Nassau, Rockland, Suffolk, and Westchester)

Return without payment:	Return with payment:
Holtsville, NY 00501-0047	P.O. Box 210
	Newark, NJ 07101-0210

New York (all other counties), Connecticut, Maine, Massachusetts, New Hampshire, Rhode Island, Vermont

Return without payment:	Return with payment:
Andover, MA 05501-0047	P.O. Box 371324
	Pittsburgh, PA 15250-7324

Illinois, Iowa, Minnesota, Missouri, Wisconsin

Return without payment:	Return with payment:
Kansas City, MO 64999-0047	P.O. Box 970010
	St. Louis, MO 63197-0010

Delaware, District of Columbia, Maryland, Pennsylvania, Puerto Rico, Virginia, U.S. Virgin Islands

Return without payment:	Return with payment:
Philadelphia, PA 19255-0047	P.O. Box 8738
	Philadelphia, PA 19162-8738

Indiana, Kentucky, Michigan, Ohio, West Virginia

Return without payment:	Return with payment:
Cincinnati, OH 45999-0047	P.O. Box 6796
	Chicago, IL 60680-6796

Kansas, New Mexico, Oklahoma, Texas

Return without payment:	Return with payment:
Austin, TX 73301-0047	P.O. Box 970017
	St. Louis, MO 63197-0017

Alaska, Arizona, California (counties of Alpine, Amador, Butte, Calaveras, Colusa, Contra Costa, Del Norte, El Dorado, Glenn, Humboldt, Lake, Lassen, Marin, Mendocino, Modoc, Napa, Nevada, Placer, Plumas, Sacramento, San Joaquin, Shasta, Sierra, Siskiyou, Solano, Sonoma, Sutter, Tehama, Trinity, Yolo, and Yuba), Colorado, Idaho, Montana, Nebraska, Nevada, North Dakota, Oregon, South Dakota, Utah, Washington, Wyoming

Return without payment:	Return with payment:
Ogden, UT 84201-0047	P.O. Box 7028
	San Francisco, CA 94120-7028

California (all other counties), Hawaii

Return without payment:	Return with payment:
Fresno, CA 93888-0047	P.O. Box 60150
	Los Angeles, CA 90060-0150

Alabama, Arkansas, Louisiana, Mississippi, North Carolina, Tennessee

Return without payment:	Return with payment:
Memphis, TN 37501-0047	P.O. Box 1210
	Charlotte, NC 28201-1210

If you have no legal residence or principal place of business in any IRS district, file with the Internal Revenue Service Center, Philadelphia, PA 19255.

Amended Returns.—Use a new Form 940-EZ to amend a previously filed Form 940-EZ. Check the Amended Return box above Part I, enter the amounts that should have been on the original return, and sign the amended return. Attach an explanation of the reasons for amending the original return.

If you were required to file Form 940 but filed Form 940-EZ instead, file the amended return on Form 940. See Form 940 and its instructions.

Specific Instructions

You must complete lines A and B and Part I. If your FUTA tax (line 6) is over $100, you must also complete Part II. Please remember to sign the return.

Line A.—Enter the dollar amount of state unemployment contributions. If your state has given you a 0% experience rate, so there are no required contributions, write "0% rate" in the space.

Part I. Taxable Wages and FUTA Tax

Line 1—Total payments.—Enter the total payments you made to employees during the calendar year, even if they are not taxable for FUTA tax. Include salaries, wages, commissions, fees, bonuses, vacation allowances, amounts paid to temporary or part-time employees, and the value of goods, lodging, food, clothing, and noncash fringe benefits. Also, include the amount of tips reported to you in writing by your employees. Enter the amount before any deductions.

How you make the payments is not important to determine if they are wages. Thus, you may pay wages for piecework or as a percentage of profits. You may pay wages hourly, daily, weekly, monthly, or yearly. You may pay wages in cash or some other way, such as goods, lodging, food, or clothing. For items other than cash, use the fair market value when paid.

Line 2—Exempt payments.—"Wages" and "employment" for FUTA purposes do not include every payment and every kind of service an employee may perform. In general, payments that are not wages and payments for services that are not employment are not subject to tax. Enter these payments here to deduct them from total payments (line 1).

Enter such items as the following:

1. Agricultural labor if you did not meet either test in **Agricultural Employers** on page 2.

2. Benefit payments for sickness or injury under a worker's compensation law.

3. Household service if you did not pay cash wages of $1,000 or more in any calendar quarter in 1993 and 1994.

4. Certain family employment.

5. Certain fishing activities.

6. Noncash payments for farmwork or household services in a private home that are included on line 1. Only cash wages to these workers are taxable.

7. Value of certain meals and lodging.

8. Cost of group-term life insurance.

9. Payments attributable to the employee's contributions to a sick-pay plan.

10. Benefits excludable under a section 125 plan (cafeteria plan).

11. Any other exempt service or pay.

For more information, see Special Rules for Various Types of Services and Products in **Circular E**, Employer's Tax Guide.

Line 3—Enter the total amounts over $7,000 you paid each employee. For example, if you have 10 employees and paid each $8,000 during the year, enter $80,000 on line 1 and $10,000 on line 3. The $10,000 is the amount over $7,000 paid to each employee. Do not include any exempt payments from line 2 in figuring the $7,000.

Part II. Record of Quarterly Federal Unemployment Tax Liability

Complete this part only if your FUTA tax on line 6 is over $100. To figure your FUTA tax liability, multiply by .008 that part of the first $7,000 of each employee's annual wages you paid during the quarter. Enter the result in the space for that quarter.

Your total liability must equal your total tax. If not, you may be charged a failure to deposit penalty.

Record your liability based on when you pay the wages, not on when you deposit the tax. For example, if you pay wages on March 29, your FUTA tax liability on those wages is $200, and you deposit the $200 by April 30, you would record that $200 in the first quarter, not the second.

Depositing FUTA Tax.—Generally, FUTA taxes are deposited quarterly. If you deposited the right amounts, following these rules, the amount you owe with Form 940-EZ will never be over $100.

Using **Form 8109**, Federal Tax Deposit Coupon, deposit FUTA tax in an authorized financial institution or the Federal Reserve bank for your area. Records of your deposits will be sent to the IRS for crediting to your business accounts.

If your liability for any of the first 3 quarters of 1994 (plus any undeposited amount of $100 or less from any earlier quarter) is over $100, deposit it by the last day of the month after the end of the quarter. If it is $100 or less, carry it to the next quarter; a deposit is not required. If your liability for the 4th quarter (plus any undeposited amount from any earlier quarter) is over $100, deposit the entire amount by January 31, 1995. If it is $100 or less, you can either make a deposit or pay it with your Form 940-EZ by January 31.

Note: *The total amount of all deposits must be shown on line 7.*

Printed on recycled paper

☆U.S. GOVERNMENT PRINTING OFFICE: 1994-375-139

Form **941**	**Employer's Quarterly Federal Tax Return**	
(Rev. April 1994) Department of the Treasury Internal Revenue Service (O)	4141 ▶ See separate instructions for information on completing this return. Please type or print.	

Enter state code for state in which deposits made ▶ [:] (see page 2 of instructions).

Name (as distinguished from trade name)	Date quarter ended	OMB No. 1545-0029
Trade name, if any	Employer identification number	T FF FD
Address (number and street)	City, state, and ZIP code	FP I T

If address is different from prior return, check here ▶ [ ]

IRS Use

1 1 1 1 1 1 1 1 1 1 2 3 3 3 3 3 3 4 4 4

5 5 5 6 7 8 8 8 8 8 8 9 9 9 10 10 10 10 10 10 10 10 '0 10

If you do not have to file returns in the future, check here ▶ [ ] and enter date final wages paid ▶

If you are a seasonal employer, see **Seasonal employers** on page 2 and check here (see instructions) ▶ [ ]

1	Number of employees (except household) employed in the pay period that includes March 12th ▶		
2	Total wages and tips subject to withholding, plus other compensation	**2**	
3	Total income tax withheld from wages, tips, and sick pay	**3**	
4	Adjustment of withheld income tax for preceding quarters of calendar year	**4**	
5	Adjusted total of income tax withheld (line 3 as adjusted by line 4—see instructions)	**5**	
6a	Taxable social security wages . . . . $ × 12.4% (.124) =	**6a**	
b	Taxable social security tips . . . . . $ × 12.4% (.124) =	**6b**	
7	Taxable Medicare wages and tips . . . . . $ × 2.9% (.029) =	**7**	
8	Total social security and Medicare taxes (add lines 6a, 6b, and 7). Check here if wages are not subject to social security and/or Medicare tax . . . . ▶ [ ]	**8**	
9	Adjustment of social security and Medicare taxes (see instructions for required explanation) Sick Pay $ _____ ± Fractions of Cents $ _____ ± Other $ _____ =	**9**	
10	Adjusted total of social security and Medicare taxes (line 8 as adjusted by line 9—see instructions)	**10**	
11	**Total taxes** (add lines 5 and 10)	**11**	
12	Advance earned income credit (EIC) payments made to employees, if any	**12**	
13	Net taxes (subtract line 12 from line 11). **This should equal line 17, column (d) below** (or line D of Schedule B (Form 941))	**13**	
14	Total deposits for quarter, including overpayment applied from a prior quarter	**14**	
15	**Balance due** (subtract line 14 from line 13). Pay to Internal Revenue Service	**15**	
16	**Overpayment,** if line 14 is more than line 13, enter excess here ▶ $ _____		

and check if to be: . [ ] Applied to next return **OR** [ ] Refunded.

- **All filers:** If line 13 is less than $500, you need not complete line 17 or Schedule B.
- **Semiweekly depositors:** Complete Schedule B and check here . . . . ▶ [ ]
- **Monthly depositors:** Complete line 17, columns (a) through (d) and check here . . . . . . ▶ [ ]

17 Monthly Summary of Federal Tax Liability.

(a) First month liability	(b) Second month liability	(c) Third month liability	(d) Total liability for quarter

Sign Here

Under penalties of perjury, I declare that I have examined this return, including accompanying schedules and statements, and to the best of my knowledge and belief, it is true, correct, and complete.

Signature ▶ | Print Your Name and Title ▶ | Date ▶

For Paperwork Reduction Act Notice, see page 1 of separate instructions.   Cat. No. 17001Z   Form **941** (Rev. 4-94)

*U.S. Government Printing Office: 1995 — 387-095/00360

9595   ☐ VOID   ☐ CORRECTED

PAYER'S name, street address, city, state, and ZIP code		1 Rents $	OMB No. 1545-0115	
		2 Royalties $	**1995**	**Miscellaneous Income**
		3 Other income $	Form **1099-MISC**	
PAYER'S Federal identification number	RECIPIENT'S identification number	4 Federal income tax withheld $	5 Fishing boat proceeds $	**Copy A** **For**
RECIPIENT'S name		6 Medical and health care payments $	7 Nonemployee compensation $	**Internal Revenue Service Center**
Street address (including apt. no.)		8 Substitute payments in lieu of dividends or interest $	9 Payer made direct sales of $5,000 or more of consumer products to a buyer (recipient) for resale ▶ ☐	**File with Form 1096.** For Paperwork Reduction Act
City, state, and ZIP code		10 Crop insurance proceeds $	11 State income tax withheld $	Notice and instructions for completing this form,
Account number (optional)	2nd TIN Not. ☐	12 State/Payer's state number		see **Instructions for Forms 1099, 1098, 5498, and W-2G.**

Form **1099-MISC**   Cat. No. 14425J   Department of the Treasury - Internal Revenue Service

Do NOT Cut or Separate Forms on This Page

9595   ☐ VOID   ☐ CORRECTED

PAYER'S name, street address, city, state, and ZIP code		1 Rents $	OMB No. 1545-0115	
		2 Royalties $	**1995**	**Miscellaneous Income**
		3 Other income $	Form **1099-MISC**	
PAYER'S Federal identification number	RECIPIENT'S identification number	4 Federal income tax withheld $	5 Fishing boat proceeds $	**Copy A** **For**
RECIPIENT'S name		6 Medical and health care payments $	7 Nonemployee compensation $	**Internal Revenue Service Center**
Street address (including apt. no.)		8 Substitute payments in lieu of dividends or interest $	9 Payer made direct sales of $5,000 or more of consumer products to a buyer (recipient) for resale ▶ ☐	**File with Form 1096.** For Paperwork Reduction Act
City, state, and ZIP code		10 Crop insurance proceeds $	11 State income tax withheld $	Notice and instructions for completing this form,
Account number (optional)	2nd TIN Not. ☐	12 State/Payer's state number		see **Instructions for Forms 1099, 1098, 5498, and W-2G.**

Form **1099-MISC**   Cat. No. 14425J   Department of the Treasury - Internal Revenue Service

Do NOT Cut or Separate Forms on This Page

9595   ☐ VOID   ☐ CORRECTED

PAYER'S name, street address, city, state, and ZIP code		1 Rents $	OMB No. 1545-0115	
		2 Royalties $	**1995**	**Miscellaneous Income**
		3 Other income $	Form **1099-MISC**	
PAYER'S Federal identification number	RECIPIENT'S identification number	4 Federal income tax withheld $	5 Fishing boat proceeds $	**Copy A** **For**
RECIPIENT'S name		6 Medical and health care payments $	7 Nonemployee compensation $	**Internal Revenue Service Center**
Street address (including apt. no.)		8 Substitute payments in lieu of dividends or interest $	9 Payer made direct sales of $5,000 or more of consumer products to a buyer (recipient) for resale ▶ ☐	**File with Form 1096.** For Paperwork Reduction Act
City, state, and ZIP code		10 Crop insurance proceeds $	11 State income tax withheld $	Notice and instructions for completing this form,
Account number (optional)	2nd TIN Not. ☐	12 State/Payer's state number		see **Instructions for Forms 1099, 1098, 5498, and W-2G.**

Form **1099-MISC**   Cat. No. 14425J   Department of the Treasury - Internal Revenue Service

Note: Self Duplicating, Carbon Paper Not Required

Form SS-8	**Determination of Employee Work Status for Purposes of Federal Employment Taxes and Income Tax Withholding**	OMB No. 1545-0004 Expires 7-31-96

Form **SS-8**
(Rev. July 1993)
Department of the Treasury
Internal Revenue Service

Paperwork Reduction Act Notice

We ask for the information on this form to carry out the Internal Revenue laws of the United States. You are required to give us this information. We need it to ensure that you are complying with these laws and to allow us to figure and collect the right amount of tax.

The time needed to complete and file this form will vary depending on individual circumstances. The estimated average time is: **recordkeeping, 34 hr., 55 min., learning about the law or the form,** 6 min. and **preparing and sending the form to IRS,** 40 min. If you have comments concerning the accuracy of these time estimates or suggestions for making this form more simple, we would be happy to hear from you. You can write to both the **Internal Revenue Service,** Attention: Reports Clearance Officer, T:FP, Washington, DC 20224; and the **Office of Management and Budget,** Paperwork Reduction Project (1545-0004), Washington, DC 20503. **DO NOT** send the tax form to either of these offices. Instead, see **General Information** for where to file.

Purpose

Employers and workers file Form SS-8 to get a determination as to whether a worker is an employee for purposes of Federal employment taxes and income tax withholding.

General Information

This form should be completed carefully. If the firm is completing the form, it should be completed for **ONE** individual who is representative of the class of workers whose status is in question. If a written determination is desired for more than one class of workers, a separate Form SS-8 should be completed for one worker from each class whose status is typical of that class. A written determination for any worker will apply to other workers of the same class if the facts are not materially different from those of the worker whose status was ruled upon.

Please return Form SS-8 to the Internal Revenue Service office that provided the form. If the Internal Revenue Service did not ask you to complete this form but you wish a determination on whether a worker is an employee, file Form SS-8 with your District Director.

Caution: Form SS-8 is not a claim for refund of social security and Medicare taxes or Federal income tax withholding. Also, a determination that an individual is an employee does not necessarily reduce any current or prior tax liability. A worker must file his or her income tax return even if a determination has not been made by the due date of the return.

Name of firm (or person) for whom the worker performed services	Name of worker
Address of firm (include street address, apt. or suite no., city, state, and ZIP code)	Address of worker (include street address, apt. or suite no., city, state, and ZIP code)

Trade name	Telephone number (include area code) ( )	Worker's social security number – –

Telephone number (include area code) ( )	Firm's taxpayer identification number –	

Check type of firm for which the work relationship is in question:
☐ **Individual**   ☐ **Partnership**   ☐ **Corporation**   ☐ **Other** (specify) ▶

Important Information Needed to Process Your Request

This form is being completed by: ☐ Firm   ☐ Worker

If this form is being completed by the worker, the IRS **must** have your permission to disclose your name to the firm.

Do you object to disclosing your name and the information on this form to the firm? . . . .   ☐ **Yes**   ☐ **No**
If you answer "Yes," the IRS cannot act on your request. **DO NOT complete the rest of this form unless the IRS asks for it.**

Under section 6110 of the Internal Revenue Code, the information on this form and related file documents will be open to the public if any ruling or determination is made. However, names, addresses, and taxpayer identification numbers must be removed before the information can be made public.

Is there any other information you want removed? . . . .   ☐ **Yes**   ☐ **No**
If you check "Yes," we cannot process your request unless you submit a copy of this form and copies of all supporting documents showing, in brackets, the information you want removed. Attach a separate statement telling which specific exemption of section 6110(c) applies to each bracketed part.

This form is designed to cover many work activities, so some of the questions may not apply to you. You must answer ALL items or mark them "Unknown" or "Does not apply." If you need more space, attach another sheet.

Total number of workers in this class. (Attach names and addresses. If more than 10 workers, attach only 10.) ▶ _____

This information is about services performed by the worker from _____ to _____
(month, day, year)   (month, day, year)

Is the worker still performing services for the firm? . . . .   ☐ **Yes**   ☐ **No**

If "No," what was the date of termination? ▶ _____
(month, day, year)

Cat. No. 16106T	Form **SS-8** (Rev. 7-93)

1a Describe the firm's business ....

b Describe the work done by the worker ....

2a If the work is done under a written agreement between the firm and the worker, attach a copy.

b If the agreement is not in writing, describe the terms and conditions of the work arrangement ....

....

c If the actual working arrangement differs in any way from the agreement, explain the differences and why they occur ....

....

3a Is the worker given training by the firm? . . . . ☐ **Yes** ☐ **No**

If "Yes": What kind? ....

How often? ....

b Is the worker given instructions in the way the work is to be done (exclusive of actual training in 3a)? . ☐ **Yes** ☐ **No**

If "Yes," give specific examples. ....

c Attach samples of any written instructions or procedures.

d Does the firm have the right to change the methods used by the worker or direct that person on how to

do the work? . . . . ☐ **Yes** ☐ **No**

Explain your answer ....

....

e Does the operation of the firm's business require that the worker be supervised or controlled in the

performance of the service? . . . . ☐ **Yes** ☐ **No**

Explain your answer ....

....

4a The firm engages the worker:

☐ To perform and complete a particular job only

☐ To work at a job for an indefinite period of time

☐ Other (explain) ....

b Is the worker required to follow a routine or a schedule established by the firm? . . . . ☐ **Yes** ☐ **No**

If "Yes," what is the routine or schedule? ....

....

c Does the worker report to the firm or its representative?. . . . . ☐ **Yes** ☐ **No**

If "Yes": How often? ....

For what purpose? ....

In what manner (in person, in writing, by telephone, etc.)? ....

Attach copies of report forms used in reporting to the firm.

d Does the worker furnish a time record to the firm?. . . . . ☐ **Yes** ☐ **No**

If "Yes," attach copies of time records.

5a State the kind and value of tools, equipment, supplies, and materials furnished by:

The firm ....

....

The worker ....

b What expenses are incurred by the worker in the performance of services for the firm? ....

....

c Does the firm reimburse the worker for any expenses? . . . . ☐ **Yes** ☐ **No**

If "Yes," specify the reimbursed expenses ....

6a Will the worker perform the services personally? . . . . ☐ **Yes** ☐ **No**

b Does the worker have helpers? . . . . ☐ **Yes** ☐ **No**

If "Yes": Who hires the helpers? ☐ Firm ☐ Worker

If hired by the worker, is the firm's approval necessary?. . . . . ☐ **Yes** ☐ **No**

Who pays the helpers? ☐ Firm ☐ Worker

Are social security and Medicare taxes and Federal income tax withheld from the helpers' wages? . . ☐ **Yes** ☐ **No**

If "Yes": Who reports and pays these taxes? ☐ Firm ☐ Worker

Who reports the helpers' incomes to the Internal Revenue Service? ☐ Firm ☐ Worker

If the worker pays the helpers, does the firm repay the worker? . . . . ☐ **Yes** ☐ **No**

What services do the helpers perform?

7   At what location are the services performed? ☐ Firm's ☐ Worker's ☐ Other (specify) ....

8a   Type of pay worker receives:
     ☐ Salary   ☐ Commission ☐ Hourly wage   ☐ Piecework ☐ Lump sum   ☐ Other (specify) ....

   b   Does the firm guarantee a minimum amount of pay to the worker? . . . . ☐ Yes   ☐ No

   c   Does the firm allow the worker a drawing account or advances against pay? . . . . ☐ Yes   ☐ No

     If "Yes": Is the worker paid such advances on a regular basis? . . . . ☐ Yes   ☐ No

   d   How does the worker repay such advances? ....

9a   Is the worker eligible for a pension, bonus, paid vacations, sick pay, etc.? . . . . ☐ Yes   ☐ No

     If "Yes," specify ....

   b   Does the firm carry workmen's compensation insurance on the worker? . . . . ☐ Yes   ☐ No

   c   Does the firm deduct social security and Medicare taxes from amounts paid the worker? . . . . . ☐ Yes   ☐ No

   d   Does the firm deduct Federal income taxes from amounts paid the worker? . . . . ☐ Yes   ☐ No

   e   How does the firm report the worker's income to the Internal Revenue Service?
     ☐ Form W-2 ☐ Form 1099-MISC ☐ Does not report ☐ Other (specify) ....
     Attach a copy.

   f   Does the firm bond the worker? . . . . ☐ Yes   ☐ No

10a   Approximately how many hours a day does the worker perform services for the firm? ....
     Does the firm set hours of work for the worker? . . . . ☐ Yes   ☐ No
     If "Yes," what are the worker's set hours? _____ am/pm to _____ am/pm (Circle whether am or pm)

   b   Does the worker perform similar services for others? . . . . ☐ Yes ☐ No ☐ **Unknown**
     If "Yes": Are these services performed on a daily basis for other firms? . . . . . . ☐ Yes ☐ No ☐ **Unknown**
     Percentage of time spent in performing these services for:
     This firm .... %   Other firms .... % ☐ **Unknown**
     Does the firm have priority on the worker's time? . . . . ☐ Yes   ☐ No
     If "No," explain ....

   c   Is the worker prohibited from competing with the firm either while performing services or during any later
     period? . . . . ☐ Yes   ☐ No

11a   Can the firm discharge the worker at any time without incurring a liability? . . . . ☐ Yes   ☐ No
     If "No," explain ....

   b   Can the worker terminate the services at any time without incurring a liability? . . . . ☐ Yes   ☐ No
     If "No," explain ....

12a   Does the worker perform services for the firm under:
     ☐ The firm's business name   ☐ The worker's own business name ☐   Other (specify) ....

   b   Does the worker advertise or maintain a business listing in the telephone directory, a trade
     journal, etc.? . . . . ☐ Yes ☐ No ☐ **Unknown**
     If "Yes," specify ....

   c   Does the worker represent himself or herself to the public as being in business to perform
     the same or similar services? . . . . ☐ Yes ☐ No ☐ **Unknown**
     If "Yes," how? ....

   d   Does the worker have his or her own shop or office? . . . . ☐ Yes ☐ No ☐ **Unknown**
     If "Yes," where? ....

   e   Does the firm represent the worker as an employee of the firm to its customers? . . . . ☐ Yes   ☐ No
     If "No," how is the worker represented? ....

   f   How did the firm learn of the worker's services? ....

13   Is a license necessary for the work? . . . . ☐ Yes ☐ No ☐ **Unknown**
     If "Yes," what kind of license is required? ....
     By whom is it issued? ....
     By whom is the license fee paid? ....

14   Does the worker have a financial investment in a business related to the services performed? ☐ Yes ☐ No ☐ **Unknown**
     If "Yes," specify and give amounts of the investment ....

15   Can the worker incur a loss in the performance of the service for the firm? . . . . ☐ Yes   ☐ No
     If "Yes," how? ....

16a   Has any other government agency ruled on the status of the firm's workers? . . . . ☐ Yes   ☐ No
     If "Yes," attach a copy of the ruling.

   b   Is the same issue being considered by any IRS office in connection with the audit of the worker's tax
     return or the firm's tax return, or has it recently been considered? . . . . ☐ Yes   ☐ No
     If "Yes," for which year(s)?

17 Does the worker assemble or process a product at home or away from the firm's place of business? . ☐ **Yes** ☐ **No**
If "Yes":
Who furnishes materials or goods used by the worker? ☐ Firm ☐ Worker
Is the worker furnished a pattern or given instructions to follow in making the product? . . . . ☐ **Yes** ☐ **No**
Is the worker required to return the finished product to the firm or to someone designated by the firm? . ☐ **Yes** ☐ **No**

Answer items 18a through n only if the worker is a salesperson or provides a service directly to customers.

18a Are leads to prospective customers furnished by the firm? . . . . ☐ **Yes** ☐ **No** ☐ **Does not apply**
b Is the worker required to pursue or report on leads? . . . . ☐ **Yes** ☐ **No** ☐ **Does not apply**
c Is the worker required to adhere to prices, terms, and conditions of sale established by the firm? . . ☐ **Yes** ☐ **No**
d Are orders submitted to and subject to approval by the firm? . . . . ☐ **Yes** ☐ **No**
e Is the worker expected to attend sales meetings? . . . . ☐ **Yes** ☐ **No**
If "Yes": Is the worker subject to any kind of penalty for failing to attend? . . . . ☐ **Yes** ☐ **No**
f Does the firm assign a specific territory to the worker? . . . . ☐ **Yes** ☐ **No** ☐ **Does not apply**
g Who does the customer pay? ☐ Firm ☐ Worker
If worker, does the worker remit the total amount to the firm? . . . . ☐ **Yes** ☐ **No**
h Does the worker sell a consumer product in a home or establishment other than a permanent retail
establishment? . . . . ☐ **Yes** ☐ **No**
i List the products and/or services distributed by the worker, such as meat, vegetables, fruit, bakery products, beverages (other than milk), or laundry or dry cleaning services. If more than one type of product and/or service is distributed, specify the principal one. ....
j Did the firm or another person assign the route or territory and a list of customers to the worker? . . ☐ **Yes** ☐ **No**
If "Yes," enter the name and job title of the person who made the assignment. ....
....
k Did the worker pay the firm or person for the privilege of serving customers on the route or in the territory? ☐ **Yes** ☐ **No**
If "Yes," how much did the worker pay (not including any amount paid for a truck or racks, etc.)? $ ....
What factors were considered in determining the value of the route or territory? ....
l How are new customers obtained by the worker? Explain fully, showing whether the new customers called the firm for service, were solicited by the worker, or both. ....
m Does the worker sell life insurance? . . . . ☐ **Yes** ☐ **No**
If "Yes":
Is the selling of life insurance or annuity contracts for the firm the worker's entire business activity? . . ☐ **Yes** ☐ **No**
If "No," list the other business activities and the amount of time spent on them ....
Does the worker sell other types of insurance for the firm? . . . . ☐ **Yes** ☐ **No**
If "Yes," state the percentage of the worker's total working time spent in selling other types of insurance .... %
At the time the contract was entered into between the firm and the worker, was it their intention that the worker sell life insurance for the firm: ☐ on a full-time basis ☐ on a part-time basis
State the manner in which the intention was expressed. ....
n Is the worker a traveling or city salesperson? . . . . ☐ **Yes** ☐ **No**
If "Yes": From whom does worker principally solicit orders for the firm? ....
If the worker solicits orders from wholesalers, retailers, contractors, or operators of hotels, restaurants, or other similar establishments, specify the percentage of the worker's time spent in this solicitation. .... %
Is the merchandise purchased by the customers for resale or for use in their business operations? If used by the customers in their business operations, describe the merchandise and state whether it is equipment installed on their premises or a consumable supply. ....

19 Attach a detailed explanation of any other reason why you believe the worker is an independent contractor or is an employee of the firm.

Under penalties of perjury, I declare that I have examined this request, including accompanying documents, and to the best of my knowledge and belief, the facts presented are true, correct, and complete.

Signature ▶   Title ▶   Date ▶

If this form is used by the firm in requesting a written determination, the form must be signed by an officer or member of the firm.
If this form is used by the worker in requesting a written determination, the form must be signed by the worker. If the worker wants a written determination about services performed for two or more firms, a separate form must be completed and signed for each firm.
Additional copies of this form may be obtained from any Internal Revenue Service office or by calling 1-800-TAX-FORM (1-800-829-3676).

*U.S. Government Printing Office: 1993 — 343-034/80171

Compliance Checklist

Carefully study the issues listed below and place a checkmark under the party you feel is responsible for each. If you are a contractor at this time, consider the way you are operating now and use that as your guide.

ISSUE	NOT APPLICABLE	SALON OWNER	CONTRACTOR
Telephone			
Cash Register			
Monies			
Retail Product			
Liability Insurance			
Business Cards			
Marketing Customers			
Promotions			
Receptionist			
Appointment Book			
Back Bar Supplies			
Station Supplies			
Chemical Products			
Small Equipment			
Large Equipment			
Sundry Products (cotton, etc.)			
Cleaning (booth/sink area, etc.)			
Cleaning Common Area (reception, bathroom, etc.)			
Meetings			
W-2 Forms			
1099 Forms			
Hiring Assistants			
Training and Advance Education			
Occupational License			

Application for Employment

Personal

Last Name	First	Middle	Date

Street Address _____ Home Telephone _____

City, State, Zip _____ Business Telephone _____

Have you ever applied for employment with us?   Pay Expected _____

❑ Yes ❑ No   If yes, Month and Year _____ Location _____

Position Desired _____   When will you be available to begin? _____

Can you attend evening meetings and/or classes? ❑ Yes ❑ No   Employment Desired:
Full Time ❑

Can you attend morning meetings and/or classes? ❑ Yes ❑ No   Part Time ❑

Can you work evenings? ❑ Yes ❑ No

Professional

(Please check applicable spaces)

1. Are you experienced in hairdressing? _____   Skin Care _____   How long? _____

2. Are you a recent beauty school graduate? _____

3. Have you worked for a nonappointment salon? _____   How long? _____

4. Special needs: Hours _____ Child Care _____ Transportation _____ Holidays _____ Insurance _____

5. I want to know about: Training _____ Benefits _____ Vacation _____ Advancement _____

Years of experience _____ Areas of specialization _____

Do you have a Cosmetology license in this state? ❑ Yes ❑ No   Type _____

Have you regularly attended any manufacturers' clinics or seminars? ❑ Yes ❑ No   Which? _____

How do you rate yourself as a hairdresser? ❑ Excellent ❑ Very Good ❑ Average ❑ Fair ❑ Poor

(Professional cont'd)

Rate the top 5 salon services you perform in order of your preference. Mark your favorite "1," your next favorite "2," etc.

☐ Cutting   ☐ Conditioning   ☐ Coloring   ☐ Styling   ☐ Other

☐ Perming   ☐ Manicuring   ☐ Skin Care   ☐ Make-up   _____

Education

School	Name and Location of School	Course of Study	No. of Years Completed	Did you Graduate?	Degree or Diploma
College				☐ Yes ☐ No	
Business/Trade/Technical				☐ Yes ☐ No	
High School				☐ Yes ☐ No	

(1)
Salon Employment

Salon Name

Telephone
(   )

Address

Employed (State month and year)
From   To

Name of Supervisor

Weekly Pay
Start   Last

State Job Title and Describe Your Work

Reason for Leaving

(2)

Salon Name

Telephone
(   )

Address

Employed (State month and year)
From   To

Name of Supervisor

Weekly Pay
Start   Last

State Job Title and Describe Your Work

Reason for Leaving

(3)

Salon Name	Telephone ( )
Address	Employed (State month and year) From To
Name of Supervisor	Weekly Pay Start Last
State Job Title and Describe Your Work	Reason for Leaving

Other Employment

(4)

Company Name	Telephone ( )
Address	Employed (State month and year) From To
Name of Supervisor	Weekly Pay Start Last
State Job Title and Describe Your Work	Reason for Leaving

References

Please list three references (include at least two professional references).

Name _____ Phone (_____) _____
Address _____
City _____ State _____ Zip Code _____
Title and/or relationship _____

Name _____ Phone (_____) _____
Address _____
City _____ State _____ Zip Code _____
Title and/or relationship _____

Name _____ Phone (_____) _____
Address _____
City _____ State _____ Zip Code _____
Title and/or relationship _____

You are required by the Immigration Reform and Control Act of 1986 to complete Form I-9 within three business days of being hired. If you are hired by this company, you must complete the form and show acceptable documentation according to Immigration and Naturalization Service guidelines. Compliance is a condition of employment.

I hereby verify that all the information I have provided on this job application is true and correct to the best of my knowledge.

Signature_____Date _____

INDEPENDENT CONTRACTOR'S AGREEMENT

THIS AGREEMENT made and entered into this _____th day of _____, by and between _____, d/b/a/ _____, hereinafter referred to as OWNER, and _____, hereinafter referred to as CONTRACTOR.

WHEREAS the parties wish to enter into an agreement by which contractor will rent certain space provided by OWNER, and

WHEREAS, CONTRACTOR intends to utilize the space provided for _____ services, and _____ and

WHEREAS, CONTRACTOR is neither an agent nor an employee of OWNER:

NOW THEREFORE, BE IT AGREED AS FOLLOWS:

1. THAT OWNER agrees to provide and CONTRACTOR agrees to rent a _____ space of the premises known as _____ .

2. THAT the initial term of this agreement shall be for _____ weeks at a rate of $_____ dollars per _____ . Either party may cancel this agreement upon two weeks' written notice. At the conclusion of the initial rental period the agreement shall continue on a month-to-month basis, or a NEW AGREEMENT shall be entered into.

3. (A) THAT the electricity, water, sinks, hooded dryers, lockable cabinets, towels, refrigerator, microwave oven, coffee maker, washer, dryer, and (optional _____) will be provided without additional charge to the CONTRAC-TOR. The CONTRACTOR agrees to conserve the electricity and water where possible. Long distance telephone service is expressly NOT provided the CON-TRACTOR under the terms of this agreement.

3. (B) Common telephone service will be provided at a monthly fee of $_____, paid separately from space rent.

4. IT IS UNDERSTOOD between the parties that OWNER is to provide CONTRACTOR only the space above described and _____ located therein. OWNER will not furnish any materials, supplies, or ingredients. CONTRACTOR expresses agrees not to contract or obligate OWNER for the purchase or payment of such supplies and agrees to indemnify her/him from liability therefore.

5. IT IS EXPRESSLY UNDERSTOOD between the parties that OWNER and his/her employees and agents shall not be responsible or liable for making CONTRAC-TOR'S appointments, receiving supplies, performing laundry services, or dealing with CONTRACTOR'S customers.

6. Any and all commercial advertisement done in the name of the salon shall be paid for equally by all CONTRACTORS. Any CONTRACTOR not wishing to participate will absolutely not be given any clients generated by the advertisements.

7. (A) THAT the space to be utilized by CONTRACTOR under the terms of this agreement shall remain the sole responsibility of the CONTRACTOR and is to be

used exclusively by the CONTRACTOR, and shall be cleaned to the owner's specifications as required by the Florida Department of Business & Professional Regulation's sanitation guidelines.

7. (B) IT IS EXPRESSLY UNDERSTOOD and agreed between the parties that the CONTRACTOR is neither an employee nor agent of _____.
Further, CONTRACTOR shall indemnify OWNER against all liability or loss, and against all claims or actions based upon or arising out of damages or injury (including death) to persons or property caused by or sustained in connection with the operations and performance of the CONTRACTOR, or by conditions created thereby, or based upon any violation of any statute, ordinance, building code, or regulation and the defense of any such claims or actions. CONTRACTOR shall also indemnify OWNER against all liability and loss in connection with and shall assume full responsibility for payment of all federal, state, and local taxes or contributions imposed or required under employment insurance, Social Security, and income tax laws with respect to any employees of the CONTRACTOR, if any.

8. CONTRACTOR agrees to furnish owner with current proof of liability and malpractice insurance coverage.

9. CONTRACTOR hereby agrees to abide by all federal and state statutes, county ordinances, and city regulations.

10. CONTRACTOR hereby agrees to be responsible for any and all damages to OWNER'S premises caused by either CONTRACTOR, his/her agents, and employees or customers.

11. (A) IF CONTRACTOR fails to comply with any of the material provisions of this agreement, other than covenant to pay rent, or materially fails to comply with any duties imposed upon the CONTRACTOR by statute, within seven (7) days after the delivery of written notice by OWNER specifying the noncompliance and indicating the intention of OWNER to terminate the agreement by reason thereof, OWNER may terminate the agreement.

11 (B) IF CONTRACTOR fails to pay rent when due and the default continues for three (3) days after delivery of written demand by OWNER for payment of the rent or possession of the premises, OWNER may terminate the agreement.

IN WITNESS WHEREOF the undersigned have hereto set their hands and seals on the day first above written.

WITNESS AS TO OWNER:

_____   _____
                                                  OWNER

_____

WITNESS AS TO CONTRACTOR:

_____   _____

_____

STATE OF FLORIDA

LEASE AGREEMENT
_____ County

This lease, made and entered into by and between
_____, hereinafter referred to as "LESSOR," and
_____, hereinafter referred to as "LESSEE,"

W I T N E S S E T H :

That Lessor does hereby lease, demise, and let unto Lessee, for use as a Hair Styling Studio, the following described premises located at _____, to-wit: A portion of _____, known as Studio _____ .
The aforementioned leased area, at the aforementioned street address, is leased upon the following terms and conditions, to-wit:

1. The duration of the lease shall commence at 12:00 A.M. on the first day of _____, and terminate on the last day of _____; however, it is agreed and understood that Lessee shall have the right to move in and occupy the demised premises at time between the execution of this lease and the specified beginning date of _____ .

2. For the initial term of this lease, the Lessee shall pay the Lessor at _____, or at any such other address as may be directed in writing from time to time by Lessor, an annual rental of _____ plus applicable sales tax payable at the rate of _____ per week plus applicable sales tax.

    All weekly rental payments (plus applicable sales tax) are due and payable in advance on Monday of each week for the duration of the lease. The first week's rent shall be due and payable in advance at time of execution of this lease.

    There shall be a late charge of six percent (6%) or the highest amount permitted under Florida law, whichever is less, levied against Lessee in event any rental payment is made five days or more after the specified due date.

3. Lessor shall pay for back bar supplies consisting of shampoo, conditioner, and towels for common use in the shampoo room. Lessor shall furnish janitorial or maid service for the common areas and trash removal and vacuum of _____ four (4) days a week. The Lessee shall, at its expense, provide for the cleaning of all the towels the lessee uses.

4. Lessor shall pay for telephone equipment and two common telephone lies. Lessee shall have access to the telephone and use of the common lines for non-toll calls.

5. Lessor shall provide furniture and furnishing for the studio, which shall include one (1) hydraulic styling chair, one (1) mirror, one (1) supply caddie, one (1) display cabinet, one (1) desk, and one (1) hair dryer. Lessee shall be responsible for the repair and upkeep of the furniture and furnishing located within Lessee's studio.

6. Lessor will provide yellow page advertising in the Tallahassee telephone book.

7. Lessor shall be responsible for the water, gas, and electrical utilities provided to and used by the studio.

8. Lessee, along with other tenants in _____, shall have the right to sue the public rest room facilities, and other common areas in _____ that Lessor has provided for its tenants.

9. Lessee hereby covenants to pay the said rent according to the terms hereof and to deliver up the premises to the Lessor peacefully and quietly at the end of the term of this lease, in

as good order and condition as presently, reasonable use and wear thereof expected.

10. The Lessee shall not assign this lease, or sublet the leased area, or any part thereof, nor use the same, or any part thereof, nor permit the same, or any part thereof, to be used for any purpose other than that as herein above indicated nor make any alterations to the demised premises, without the prior written consent of the Lessor. All additions, and all fixtures or improvements, which may be made by the Lessee, except movable fixtures, movable improvements, movable tables, chairs, displays, wares, merchandise, and office furniture and furnishings, shall become the property of the Lessor and remain upon and within the leased part thereof, and be surrendered with the leased area at the termination of the lease.

11. All personal property placed or moved in the leased area above described shall be at the risk of the Lessee or owners thereof, and Lessor shall not be liable for any damage to said personal property, or to the Lessee, the Lessee's employees, agents, licensees, or invitee, or to the Lessee's business, arising out of any act or omission of any other Lessees or occupants of the building or of any other person whomsoever, unless such damage shall be proximately caused by an act or omission of Lessor.

12. The Lessee shall promptly comply with all statutes, ordinances, rules, orders, regulations, and requirements of the Federal, State, County, and City governments and of any and all their departments and Bureaus applicable to said premises, for the correction, prevention, and abatement of nuisances or other grievances with Lessee's control, in, upon, or connected with said leased area during the said term.

13. Lessee shall not attach, apply, or affix any sign, poster, lettering, or other device or structure in or about the leased area or in or upon the Building that is visible in the Building or is visible from the streets, sidewalks, and other public areas adjoining the building without first obtaining the written consent of the Lessor. Such approval shall not be unreasonably withheld.

14. In the event the leased premises become untenantable because of damage by fire or other casualty and the leased premises cannot be restored to a tenantable condition within ninety (90) days, Lessee, at its option, can terminate this lease and shall have no further liability for rent after date of casualty and a prorata share of any rent paid in advance shall be returned to Lessee. If the leased premises can be made tenantable within ninety (90) days or if the Lessee does not elect to terminate the lease, the rent shall be abated for the period the leased premises remain untenantable.

   In the event the leased premises are damaged by fire or other casualty, but not to such extent as to make them untenantable, the leased premises shall be promptly restored to proper condition by Lessor and a just proportionate part of the rent according to the nature and extent of the damage sustained shall be abated until the premises have been duly repaired by the Lessor.

   All repairs made by Lessor shall be in conformity with all applicable Federal, State, and Local laws and ordinances and shall be made in such manner and design as to allow Lessee to continue to operate their business.

15. If the Lessee shall abandon or vacate the leased area before the end of the term of this lease, or shall suffer the rent to be in arrears, the Lessor may, at its option, forthwith cancel this lease or may enter said leaded area as the agent of the Lessee,

by force or otherwise, without being liable in any way, therefore, and relet the leased area with or without any furniture that may be therein, as the agent of the Lessee, at such price and upon such terms and for such duration of time as the Lessor may determine, and receive the rent, therefore, applying the same payment of the rent due by these presents, and if the full rental herein shall not be realized by Lessor over and above the expenses to Lessor in such re-letting, the said Lessee shall pay any deficiency, and if more than the full rental is realized, Lessor will pay over to said Lessee the excess on demand.

16. Lessee agrees to pay the cost of collection and reasonable attorney's fees in the event Lessor commences action in any court for possession of the leased area, for collection of rent or for damage to the leased area or to other tenants, or for breach of this lease by Lessee.

17. The Lessor, or any of its agents, shall have the right to enter said leased area during all reasonable hours, upon reasonable notice to Lessee or their agents, to examine the leased area, to make such repairs, additions, or alterations as may be deemed necessary for the safety, comfort, or preservation thereof of said building, or to exhibit said leased areas. The right shall likewise exist for the purpose of removing placards, signs, fixture, alterations, or additions which do not conform to this agreement or to the rules and regulations of the building.

18. Lessee agrees to maintain said leased area in the same condition, order, and repair as it is at the commencement of said term, excepting only reasonable wear and tear arising from the use thereof under this agreement, and to make good to said Lessor immediately upon demand any damage to electrical lights or fixtures, appliances, or appurtenances of said leased area, or of the building, caused by actor neglect of

Lessee, or of any person or persons in the employ of or upon the premises of or under control of the Lessee or at Lessee's invitation.

19. If the Lessee shall become insolvent or if bankruptcy proceedings shall be begun by or against the Lessee before the end of said term, the Lessor is irrevocably authorized at its option to forthwith cancel this lease, as for default. Lessor may elect to accept rent from such receiver, trustee, or other judicial officer during the term of their occupancy in their fiduciary capacity without affecting the Lessor's rights as contained in this contract, but no receiver, trustee, or other judicial officer shall ever have any right, title, or interest in or to the above described property by virtue of this contract.

20. In regard to potential liens that might be filed pursuant to Chapter 713, Florida Statutes, the parties hereby agree, in accordance with Section 713.10, that the leased premises shall not be subject to liens or claims that might result from Lessee making improvements on the demised premises.

21. Any notice to the Lessor shall be given in writing by certified mail at _____, and any notice to Lessee shall be given in writing by certified mail to_____ . Either party may designate in writing a different address for the giving of such notice.

22. The Lessor assumes no responsibility for insuring the contents of the leased area and assumes no liability for any injury or damage not proximately caused by any act or omission of the Lessor.

23. Lessee agrees to indemnify and hold harmless against all claims, demands, damages, costs, and expenses, including reasonable attorney's fees for the defense thereof, arising

from the conduct or management of Lessee's business in the leased premises or from any breach on the part of the Lessee of any conditions in this lease, or from any act or negligence of Lessee or its agents, contractors, employees, sublessees, concessionaires, or licenses in or about the leased premises. In case of any action or proceeding brought against Lessor by reason of such claim, Lessee, upon notice from Lessor, covenants to defend such action or proceeding by counsel acceptable to Lessor.

24. Time is the essence of this contract and in all its terms and conditions.

25. This lease contains the entire agreement between the parties and shall not be modified in any manner except by the parties or their respective successors in this lease and shall bind and inure to the benefit of Lessor and Lessee and their respective successors and assigns.

26. All tenants within the building of which the leased premises are a part use the same HVAC system circulating air to all parts of the building. A majority of the tenants have requested that the entire building be designated as "smoke-free." Tenants agree to implement such policies and rules as shall be necessary to implement this smoke-free policy.

IN WITNESS WHEREOF, the parties have hereunto set their hands and seals this _____ day of _____, 19____.

Witnesses as to Lessor:

_____   BY: _____
                                           (Partner)

_____

Witnesses as to Lessee:

_____

                                    _____
_____   (Lessee)

Index

employee council, 85
employee empowerment, 80
employee etiquette, 47
Employee's Withholding
    Allowance Certificate (Form
    W-4), 123-24
employees, 90
Employer Identification
    Number application (Form
    SS-4), 119-22
Employer's Quarterly Federal
    Tax Return (Form 941), 132
employment application, 4-5,
    24-30, 139-41
Employment Eligibility
    Verification (Form I-9), 125-
    26
employment qualifications, 48
energetic employees, 70
evaluations and reviews, 50

F

Federal Unemployment Tax
    Return (Form 940), 128-31
fifty five % productivity, 115
firing employees, 24
flexibility, 81

G

gossiping, 51
government forms, 116-18
gross profit, 107

H

high touch, 83
hiring, 21, 80. *See also* inter-
    view

customer concept, 33-35
determining needs of,
    7-10
effective techniques, 4
employment application,
    24-30
faulty techniques, 3-4
motivating staff, 30-31
recruiting ideas, 22-23

I

independent contractor agree-
    ment, 142-43
independent contractors, 91-94
influencing personalities, 12-
    15
internal assessments, 84
Internal Revenue Service, 88-
    99
interview, 4-5, 37
        guidelines for, 38-39
        questions for applicant,
            39-41
        statement of salon
    owner's needs, 41-43

J

jealousy, 71
job descriptions, 43, 47-48

L

labor and product costs, 107
lease agreement, 144-50
lost employees, 84
loyalty, 80
lunch and break policy, 50

Notes

Style.
Savvy.
Solutions.

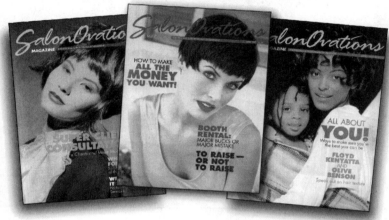

every month.
SalonOvations

SalonOvations is a professional and personal magazine designed with you in mind. Each issue delivers great features on personal growth and on-target stories about the beauty business. Get helpful hints from industry pros on starting your own salon business and how to satisfy your clients. Plus, you'll get pages of colorful photos of the latest trends in haircutting, styling and coloring.

All this at a great price of 12 **15** issues for only $19.95 a year! **3 FREE issues** - Save over 40%

(price subject to change)